The Family in Medical Practice
A Family Systems Primer

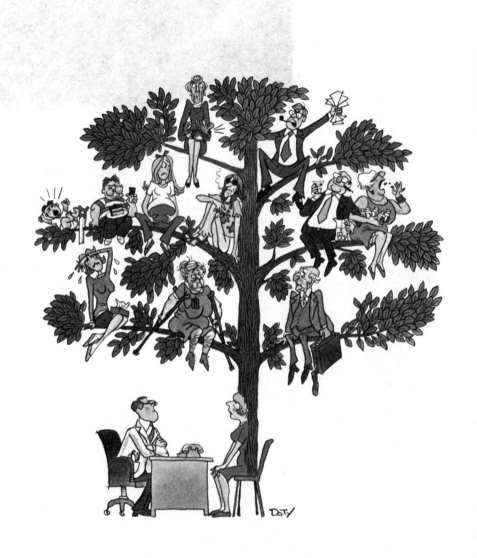

The Family
in Medical Practice
A Family Systems Primer

Edited by
Michael A. Crouch and Leonard Roberts

With 29 Figures

Springer-Verlag
New York Berlin Heidelberg
London Paris Tokyo

MICHAEL A. CROUCH, M.D., M.S.P.H.
Department of Family Medicine and Comprehensive Care, Louisiana State University School of Medicine, Shreveport, Louisiana 71130, U.S.A.

LEONARD ROBERTS, M.D.
Department of Psychiatry, University of Rochester, Rochester, New York 14642, U.S.A.

Permission to reprint illustrations has been provided as follows:
p. ii, Roy Doty/*Patient Care*. © 1974, Patient Care Communications, Inc., Darien, CT. All rights reserved; p. 2, © 1982, Cowles Syndicate, Inc. All rights reserved; p. 14, © 1983, George Dole/*Medical Economics;* p. 23, © Cowles Syndicate, Inc. All rights reserved; p. 176, © 1985, Filchok/*Hospital Tribune;* p. 178, © 1972, Cowles Syndicate, Inc. All rights reserved.

Library of Congress Cataloging in Publication Data
The family in medical practice.
  Includes bibliographies and index.
  1. Family medicine. 2. Family—Health and hygiene.
3. Family psychotherapy. I. Crouch, Michael A.
II. Roberts, Leonard, M.D. III. Title: Family systems
primer. [DNLM: 1. Family. 2. Family Practice.
WB 110 F1937]
R729.5.G4F34 1986 610   86-13111

Typeset by David E. Seham Associates Inc., Metuchen, New Jersey.
Printed and bound by R.R. Donnelley & Sons Co., Harrisonburg, Virginia.
Printed in the United States of America.

9 8 7 6 5 4 3 2 1

ISBN 0-387-96372-3 Springer-Verlag New York Berlin Heidelberg
ISBN 3-540-96372-3 Springer-Verlag Berlin Heidelberg New York

*To the families from whence we came, and
to the families we have been fortunate enough to join,
personally and professionally*

Foreword

My practice life has spanned 36 years and during that time I have been involved in untangling countless mysterious maladies—or at least trying to do so. All of these efforts were without the benefit of any formal training about family systems. I am greatly encouraged by this book because it first draws attention to the intricate web that mankind has woven for itself. The family physician has often been caught up in this web, and therefore rendered impotent. Efforts to understand all of this are to be applauded.

It has been my good fortune to know the editors, Leonard Roberts and Michael Crouch and, as a family physician, I feel that their "hearts are in the right place." They have grown up, medically speaking, in an era when society has become more complex, where life is not easy. Birth and its medical participants are suspect; childhood is complicated by divorce and loneliness; adolescence is a time of aimless searching; young adults are hard pressed to earn a living; the quality of life is being threatened somewhat by the overgrowth of high technology; dying with dignity is at a premium. The editors are to be commended for helping us clarify the role of the family physician in all of this.

To have some system to figure out a way to find the possible pleasure that can come from getting in the boat with a troubled family, picking up an oar, and helping them to find peace, is a very special gift. This book invites us all into such a world. It does not take the place of wounds and the scars that come from the healing of the wounds of every day practice, but it offers structure and guidance. The cases presented here came from real life. This is not fiction. After all, family practice has nothing to do with that which is fictitious.

I believe that the only ingredient missing from these pages is you. Read them and create your own special brand of magic.

B. Lewis Barnett, Jr., M.D.
Charlottesville

Preface

Clinicians and scholars in several disciplines have developed theories and clinical methods for addressing how the family interacts with the health and illness of the individual. No particular family theory is widely acknowledged as the most useful way to help individuals and families with their problems. With advocates of various approaches all vigorously promoting their views, it can be difficult for the health care practitioner to decide which concepts and perspectives to use in developing practical clinical skills.

Systems theory is a general way of thinking about the world. It departs from simplistic everyday logic and reasoning. Thinking about patients and their families as interrelated elements in complex systems can usefully augment the clinician's pragmatic commonsense approaches. The authors of this book present principles from several family systems theories and illustrate how they can be applied in medical practice. The approaches covered in most detail are (in order of decreasing emphasis) multigenerational (Bowen and Satir), structural (Minuchin), problem-oriented (Doherty and Baird), and strategic (Haley).

Customized vocabularies are developed by experts to communicate with each other within specific fields of knowledge. This book explains special terms by focusing on their meanings and clinical implications, rather than on the jargon itself. Analagous terms are either used as synonyms or are differentiated by subtle differences. The Glossary of Terms further clarifies some closely related terms.

Some of the authors incorporate humor into their discussion of serious family issues because they believe humor to be an integral part of a healthy individual's life and an essential ingredient of a vibrant family life. Just as an individual benefits from taking him/herself seriously, but not overly so, the health professional can help families by regarding their issues earnestly without losing sight of the irony and levity that pervade even families with grave problems. Humor can be one of the clinician's most useful therapeutic tools when used thoughtfully and respectfully.

Reading this book will hopefully help health professionals take better care of their patients by dealing more effectively with the family aspects of their problems. The intended audience includes: students and teachers of medicine, nursing, social work, psychology, and allied health fields; resident physicians in family practice, psychiatry, pediatrics and medicine; and established health care professionals interested in learning more about family-oriented approaches to helping people.

Although the chapters are interrelated and arranged in a logical sequence, the content of each chapter stands on its own, and chapters may be easily read in any desired order. Chapters 1–5 present current knowledge about the family and health care. Chapters 6–8 explain practical skills for working with families clinically. Chapter 9 encourages the reader to grow personally and professionally by studying his/her own family. Chapter 10 previews future developments in family-oriented medical practice, research, and education.

The editors are grateful to their secretaries, Lillian Irving and Barbara Tuttle, for their invaluable assistance, to the authors for their diligence and patience, and to the staff at Springer-Verlag for their unwavering support and professionalism. We would greatly appreciate feedback from the readers about the usefulness and limitations of the book, and we welcome suggestions on how to improve the next edition.

July 30, 1986   Michael A. Crouch
                                                 Leonard Roberts

Contents

Contributors

LISA BAKER, PH.D., Assistant Professor, Department of Family Medicine, Health Sciences Center, University of Oklahoma, Oklahoma City, Oklahoma, U.S.A.

THOMAS CAMPBELL, M.D., Assistant Professor, Departments of Family Medicine and Psychiatry, University of Rochester, Rochester, New York, U.S.A.

JANET CHRISTIE-SEELY, M.D., Associate Professor, Department of Family Medicine, University of Ottawa, Ottawa, Ontario, Canada

MICHAEL A. CROUCH, M.D., M.S.P.H., Assistant Professor, Department of Family Medicine and Comprehensive Care, Louisiana State University School of Medicine at Shreveport; Medical Director, Family Practice Center; Associate Director, Family Practice Residency Program, Shreveport, Louisiana, U.S.A.

TERRY DAVIS, PH.D., Clinical Assistant Professor, Department of Family Medicine and Comprehensive Care, Louisiana State University School of Medicine at Shreveport; Coordinator, Behavioral Science Training, Family Practice Residency Program, Shreveport, Louisiana, U.S.A.

KAREN KINGSOLVER, PH.D., Department of Family Medicine, University of Washington, Renton, Washington, U.S.A.

SUSAN MCDANIEL, PH.D., Assistant Professor, Departments of Family Medicine and Psychiatry, University of Rochester, Rochester, New York, U.S.A.

LEONARD ROBERTS, M.D., Department of Psychiatry, University of Rochester, Rochester, New York, U.S.A.

HOWARD F. STEIN, PH.D., Professor, Department of Family Medicine, Health Sciences Center, University of Oklahoma, Oklahoma City, Oklahoma, U.S.A.

KAREN WEIHS, M.D., Department of Psychiatry, William S. Middleton Memorial Veterans' Hospital, Madison, Wisconsin, U.S.A.

CHAPTER 1

The History of the Family in Medicine

Janet Christie-Seely and Michael A. Crouch

Why the Family?

The family is the missing piece of the medical puzzle. In the past two decades, physicians have become increasingly frustrated by the discrepancies between what they see patients for and what they were trained to expect. The pure biomedical model of illness taught in medical school applies to only about 20% of what primary care physicians see in their offices (1). About 35% of visits involve mainly psychosocial problems, and another 35% are for self-limited illness for which little treatment is necessary or effective. The remaining 10% of visits are for prevention (e.g., checkups, well child care).

In the history of science, when old traditional concepts are no longer adequate, the time is ripe for a paradigm shift—a revision of the prevailing way of explaining something in the universe (2). Several intellectual leaders in medicine have stated that a new way of thinking about illness is needed (2–5). Medicine is now in the first stage of making a shift in understanding. This chapter will outline some of the reasons for the change, and discuss some of the ways medicine is changing. The remainder of the book will examine the detailed implications of thinking in a different way about patients than most 20th-century physicians were trained to think.

The Biomedical Model and Ambulatory Patients

Physicians have always felt inadequately prepared by their education to deal with the typical dilemmas of practice. One physician complained, for example: "People come in with persistent physical complaints which I cannot explain. Others come in, apparently wanting to be pronounced healthy; but when this is done, they become upset and appear to want a diagnosis of some clearcut physical illness instead which could explain their distress to them and to their families. Other people come in repeatedly for medical appointments, but it is not clear to me why they come, why they keep coming back and what they want from me. It is as if I am supposed to discover why they continue seeking my attention" (6).

When the physician inquires about the patient's life circumstances, many apparently straightforward episodes of illness turn out to stem from some disturbance of the patient's relationship with the social environment (7). More individuals in the community have symptoms or illness, but do not visit a doctor, than the ones who come to doctors' offices (8). Minor symptoms may push the patient beyond his/her limit of tolerance and prompt him/her to visit the doctor seeking relief if he/she is also under stress at work or at home. The symptom may be presented as a "ticket of admission" to get help for relationship problems at home or work. Unfortunately, adults ask straightforwardly for what they want less easily than the child in the cartoon who wants a hug.

Exacerbations of chronic illness are often related to changes at home. Much evidence indicates that stress can aggravate or precipitate serious "organic disease" (9). Widows or widowers have at least double the normal mortality rate for their age from cancer, heart disease, tuberculosis, and pneumonia during the first year after the death of their spouses (10).

Three brief cases from the first author's practice illustrate how the biomedical model is often inadequate. Understanding disease, recognizing its first signs, and knowing appropriate medical treatments are essential for all physicians. This understanding alone, however, is insufficient for taking good care of many patients. Understanding the broader issues in-

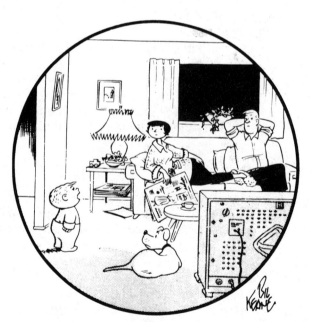

"I don't feel so good. I think I need a hug."

volved is especially important for family physicians, general internists, pediatricians, and psychiatrists, and will facilitate better outcomes for surgeons and medical subspecialists (11).

Clinical Example #1

Mrs. S, a 35-year-old pathology technician, came to see her physician with a variety of symptoms: hirsutism, a milky discharge from her breasts, fatigue, headaches, and irregular menses. She had no changes in vision, weight loss, or other systemic or focal symptoms. An endocrine problem, primarily a pituitary adenoma, had to be ruled out.

Patients sometimes keep visiting their doctors until they have provided the doctors with an adequate set of symptoms to prompt inquiry into a specific disease or syndrome (12). This lady had come with minor complaints before, but this set of symptoms spurred the physician into action. A skull film showed what was feared, a questionable double contour of the sella turcica. Hormone levels were all normal, however. After some further testing, an endocrinologist pronounced her healthy. It was then that Mrs. S broke down and described her recent stresses.

Her husband had von Recklinghausen's disease; multiple tumors had produced deafness, blindness, and mental changes. He was now institutionalized because he was extremely paranoid and dangerous to himself and his wife. He had narrowly escaped dying when he plunged a kitchen knife several inches into his chest, after announcing she was trying to poison him. Her parents, rather than understanding her predicament and supporting her wish to get a divorce and remarry, stated that she should be a good wife to him until the end. She visited him daily despite his abuse, but very much wanted a new life for herself and her 7-year-old son.

She eventually became suicidal. At that point her physician suggested meeting with Mrs. S and her parents, who lived several hundred miles away. To her surprise, her parents came, and the family communicated in a way they had never been able to do before. Mrs. S described her feelings of loneliness and desperation. Her parents talked about their wish to help her by maintaining old values. In the discussion the parents recognized that their well-intended attempts to help had actually hurt the patient, as well as her brother, whose problems they had handled similarly. They subsequently changed their relationship with the patient and her brother. The unwritten family rule that feelings should not be expressed was broken—permanently. Mrs. S stopped having suicidal thoughts and physical symptoms, and remains healthy several years later.

Clinical Example #2

Mrs. E, age 24, had frequent colds one spring. On her umpteenth visit, the physician asked her how things were at home. She began to cry, and said that raising two small children with little help from her husband was very difficult. She was encouraged to come back, together with her husband, to explore the situation more fully.

During the next visit a genogram was done to record the family relationships and dates of stresses. (See Chapter 8 for details of this technique.) Mr. E's father had died in January of the current year. Mr. E had had symptoms of arthritis two years before, when he lost his job. [Unemployment is associated with a 41% incidence of joint swelling, accompanied by some biochemical changes (13).] A week after his father died, he again began to have joint swelling and fever, and a week later was admitted to the hospital with acute rheumatoid arthritis. The couple was of the "stiff upper lip" variety and had never discussed their stresses. Mr. E had cried a little after his father's death, but in private. He had not mourned in front of the children or his wife. Avoiding open discussion of his understandably intense emotions appeared to play a key role in the emergence of a physical illness to which he was predisposed. It also generated tension in the couple, which they both tried to ignore.

In medical practice, the clinician who asks about recent deaths and how people have mourned them very frequently finds that physical illness and family dysfunction follow the death. The physician who talks with family members and encourages them to talk with each other about their feelings around the time of a death can help prevent such morbidity (14,15).

Clinical Example #3

The first author followed Mr. and Mrs. F in her practice for 8 years, observing that they alternated in the sick role. For several months the wife would come with severe arthritis, for which she tried many medications. Then the husband would present with depression for several months. When he was symptomatic, she would be relatively symptom free, and vice versa. They did not respond when this seesaw of symptoms was commented on. Only after a daughter left for Australia, and Mr. F became severely depressed, did the couple admit to stresses in the family. They were referred to a multiple family therapy group.

Apparently Mr. F, a very pleasant man, could not say no to any request when he was well. When he was depressed, however, he was able to get out of jobs given him by his wife, his church, and the community. Mrs. F was also an agreeable person, but when her arthritis acted up she was unable to do work around the house as her husband requested. Symptoms served as a means of saying no for both of them.

A more important piece of background information was that the wife had lost two brothers, who committed suicide. She was terrified that her husband would kill himself too. This she never openly acknowledged, but prior to the family therapy she panicked at the first signs of depressed mood in Mr. F, and proceeded to take meticulous care of him. (She also worked as a nurse, so she was well trained as a caretaker.) She restricted his activities and generally controlled him. In response, his depression would nosedive until her arthritis flared up and she backed off. This history fits with previous descriptions of the input of a spouse into depression (16,17).

After several months of therapy, Mrs. F's arthritis essentially disappeared. Mr. F's depressions became minor mood swings, and he was able to stop seeing the psychiatrist with whom he had been in individual-oriented psychotherapy. Open discussion of her grief for her brothers, and for her father, who died when she was 9, contributed to Mrs. F's resolving some long-standing conflicts.

The Biomedical Model and Hospitalized Patients

Even in large teaching hospitals where "organic" disease predominates, about one-fourth of all patients may be misdiagnosed because of insufficient knowledge about family factors such as the anniversary reaction (symptoms occurring around the same time of year as the death of a relative, often mimicking the dead person's symptoms).

Frequent hospital admissions for labile diabetic children, and for severe asthma, often reflect family tension (18). Typically these children become symptomatic at home, but are easily controlled in the hospital. One diabetic child, for example, was not controlled with 150 units of insulin in 15 hours at home, but was well controlled with only 30 units in 24 hours while in the hospital (19). Family therapy has reduced the hospitalization rate dramatically for children both with asthma and with diabetes.

Clinical Example #4: Heart Disease and Family Turmoil

In one study 75% of admissions for congestive heart failure followed an acute family crisis (20). The first author has a patient, Mary M, now aged 62, who exemplifies this connection between psychosocial stress and physiologic decompensation.

Mary had been hospitalized an average of three times a year for 20 years for congestive heart failure or ventricular tachycardia. Her first admission followed her onset of high blood pressure soon after one of her sons was stillborn.

Questioning about family patterns revealed that hospital admissions sometimes occurred after dramatic temper outbursts by a manic-depressive daughter. The daughter was still home at age 35, as was a 32-year-old son. (See Figure 1.1 for genogram. Chapter 8 explains genograms in detail.)

Evidence of delayed development and failed maturation in children usually reflects problems in the couple relationship. This couple had many conflicts, one of which involved sex. The wife slept in the sitting room because she could not manage the stairs. The lack of privacy and the presence of son and daughter protected her from her husband's sexual advances most of the time. Her husband's occasional insistence on having intercourse was another trigger for hospitalization.

Mary also admitted that she sometimes got exhausted at home and needed a rest in the hospital. Her role at home was that of peacemaker, ostensibly protecting her husband from the two explosive children still at home and the two others who visited frequently. She commented that when she was in the hospital, she felt like a queen and "everyone worships me." Positive attention from health professionals is often an acceptable substitute for scarce or nonexistent favorable attention from family members. Mary learned the sick role from her mother, who had avoided

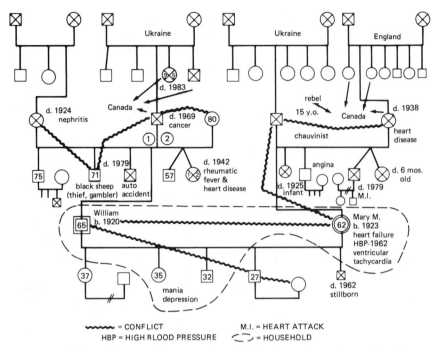

FIGURE 1.1.   Family genogram revealing ventricular tachycardia and family explosions as coevolving phenomena.

battling with Mary's angry and domineering father by going into the hospital, also with heart disease. Her mother died when Mary was 15, and, according to Mary, welcomed death.

Mary's husband William also had a family history of heart disease. When he was 22, his sister Marie, who had had rheumatic fever, died at age 12 after a long illness in which he was her main caretaker and financial support. Her death reminded him of the death of their mother, who had died when he was 4 years old. He had repressed the trauma of this early loss, but was now reliving it and the loss of his sister every time his wife was admitted to the hospital. The admissions had always occurred after he stayed home from work to look after Mary. Escalating anxiety on both their parts appeared to trigger her episodes of arrhythmia and cardiac decompensation, probably through increased catecholamine levels.

After 4 months of family therapy, the two adult children moved out of the home. Sexual relations were reestablished, since there was now privacy and Mary had begun working through her Victorian edicts against female sexuality. It has now been over a year since her last admission. The couple is planning a trip to Florida, with the cardiologist's blessing, something they could not have contemplated before. Mary and her husband both had to mourn their mothers' deaths. Their families' failure to mourn adequately when they were children had blocked emotional expression ever since.

This family's experience is not unusual. If a physician takes the time to understand family members' reactions to illness and death, and to identify the secondary gains or payoffs of illness, such complex interrelationships between family dynamics and disease often emerge.

Historical Perspective

The time is now ripe for a coordinated attack on the problems of family adjustment in relation to the maintenance of health and the treatment of illness. (21)

The above quote might easily have come from the past decade, but in fact it was written in 1945 by Henry Barber Richardson, an internist and psychiatrist, reporting on a study that will be discussed later in the chapter.

The modern history of the family in medicine involves three parallel developments that are now converging. The first was physicians and other health professionals recognizing that the patient's family context strongly influences health and illness. The second was family therapists developing a body of theory about families, beginning in the 1950s. The third development was family medicine, which arose in response to public and professional dissatisfaction with the increasingly fragmented, technocratic, and episodic nature of medical care.

Family medicine's focus on comprehensive and continuous care for the whole person, rather than just disease, led naturally to an interest in the person's immediate social environment. The family has been treated as an important unit of care by many general practitioners who were the family doctors in the past. This appreciation has been revived by the specialty of family practice, and has been reinforced by family theories borrowed from the discipline of family therapy.

Galen, Hippocrates, and Osler, among others, clearly realized that psychosocial factors influenced disease. Until recently, the impact of psychic stress on the body was a clinical observation, unconfirmed by research. The family doctor of the past, revered for his care and concern for the whole family, was also well aware of the interrelationship of psyche and soma. Although he had few effective medications, he used himself well as a therapeutic instrument, or as "the drug, doctor" (12). Although research has since clarified pathophysiology and treatment, and has greatly increased the number and usefulness of available therapies, the therapeutic use of self is still one of the physician's most valuable treatment modalities.

In 1910, the Flexner Report triggered extensive reorganization in medical education (22), resulting in reformed standards and longer training. Many of the schools that served as "diploma mills," producing large numbers of general practitioners (albeit poorly trained), were closed down by the ensuing Flexnerian purge. Raising educational standards was laudable, but somehow in the reshuffling of priorities, the medical profession gradually lost sight of the public need and desire for family-oriented health care. Particularly after World War II, knowledge and technology increased rapidly, and great advances were made in medical care. In the process, however, most medical leaders became fascinated with ever-more-dazzling technology, and lost touch with the primacy of the doctor–patient relationship.

During the same time, physicians gravitated away from functioning as generalists and toward increasingly narrow subspecialties. This was an understandable response to the rapid growth in knowledge: "Since it is obviously impossible to know it all, I will pick out a manageable area to master and with which to keep up." It is one adaptive way to handle the discomfort of uncertainty. As result of these trends, however, physicians focused more on disease, and less on the patient—more on what could be measured in the lab, and less on the seemingly unpredictable human side of medicine.

During this time, there were isolated islands of physicians who recognized the limitations of the emerging biomedical model and did something about it. In 1926, a "family club" was opened in a small house in southeast London, England (23). This enterprise was conceived as a community center in which activities would be encouraged and health care provided. The unit of care was the family, and the center was a "living laboratory" in which to observe families and promote healthy living (5). This research project used the methods of anthropology, and Margaret Mead was one of the advisers. She was married to Gregory Bateson at the time, who was later one of the first to write about family systems theory.

After three years it became the Pioneer Health Centre, with 112 families, a new building, swimming pool, gymnasium, music room, library and quiet room, nursery, dance floor, theatre, cafeteria and club, outdoor grounds, a store, and consulting rooms for physicians. The physicians performed a "periodic health overhaul" on each family once a year, and focused more on health than on illness. In 1939 it was clear to the 1400 families involved "that the best way to improve individual health was to strengthen the family through providing opportunities for growth and self-care within the wider social and physical environment" (5). Because of the onset of World War II, the project had to be closed.

An endeavor similar to the Pioneer Health Centre was the Macey Foundation's study of the family and health care, beginning in New York in 1933. Also influenced by Margaret Mead, this study was based on a model of the "family as organism" (5). In his report on the project (*Patients Have Families*), Richardson observed that illness, particularly chronic illness, can become part of family homeostasis (21). Chronic illness can be maintained by the family, who may thwart efforts of the medical profession, and sometimes of the patient, to cure the illness. Richardson also observed that medical charting and attitudes toward interviewing often obscure obvious interrelationship. For example, "the death of a relative may appear on one page and the date of the onset of the patient's symptoms on two pages below, so that there is no reason to suspect that that both events occurred in the same week" (21).

The way data are stated can also obscure interrelationships. "It is customary, for instance, to state the age of parent at death, and not the patient's age at the time, although often the latter is much the more important for the understanding of the illness" (21). In the patient with rheumatoid arthritis described earlier, his chart recorded only that his father had died at 65, not that the death was in January and immediately preceded the patient's symptoms.

Richardson also observed the effect of the medical model on the public: "Misconceptions on the part of the medical profession, like the dichotomy of mind and body, are absorbed by the general public and continue to haunt the scene, no matter how vigorously the ghost is exorcised" (21). The concept of functional or psychosomatic illness versus physical or organic illness is useful for describing the presence or absence of detectable tissue changes in the body, but the terms have perpetuated the false mind–body dualism.

After World War II, a second project in New York, the Family Health Maintenance Demonstration Project, studied 100 families matched and compared with an equal number of controls (24). Unfortunately the study designers based their data collection and analysis on an individual intrapsychic orientation, so that observations of the effects of family interactions on illness were minimal.

At the time these projects were underway, little research supported the underlying ideas. Since then considerable research has provided a firm base for looking at the family as an important source of health and illness. As result, Engel has stated the need for a new medical model—a biopsychosocial model that addresses all the pertinent dimensions of an individual's life that relate to his/her health, including the family, the community, and the workplace (3). Much research indicates that, in one sense, all illness is psychosomatic, in that it always has both psychic and somatic components. It no longer makes sense to say that the physician is caretaker for physical illness only, and the problems of living that lead to and from it are not his/her domain.

In 1970 Kuhn outlined the structure of scientific revolutions (2). To explain the world, science develops a series of abstractions and laws, which in turn determine the further questions scientists ask. As more and more new observed phenomena fail to fit the predictions of the old abstractions, the conventional theory gives way to new theory. The yielding of the old ideas is not a smooth process, however, with proponents defending the old dogma from attack by the new thinkers. Such a dramatic "paradigm shift" occurred when Einstein revolutionized the old Newtonian physics. The old view was reductionistic (one cause and one effect), and it was linear (cause A leading straight to result B). The new scientific way of thinking was cybernetic (multiple units interrelating with each other bidirectionally, e.g., mass and energy) and interactive (units affecting each other interdependently, e.g., time and space).

Biology and ecology are now based on cybernetic or systems thinking. The world is perceived as a series of increasingly larger units, one within the next in a hierarchy of systems (25) (see Figure 1.2). The same governing principles apply to each system level, whether it be a cell, organ, individual, family, or community system. Medicine has applied these principles at the cellular and organ system level, but has been slow to recognize the interactional nature of disease in the social context. It has retained a reductionistic, mechanistic view of the etiology of disease, like Newtonian physics. Unfortunately, when variables are isolated from the environment, the total reality of the phenomenon is lost in the extraction process.

The experimental method has worked very well for discovering some of the causal agents of disease, especially infectious agents. It has also led to therapeutic interventions that are usually very effective. These gains have been at the expense of the clarity of the total picture. The sharp focus on disease in the foreground leaves the patient in the distant background as an indistinct blur. Some of the time, disease can be treated with this approach and the patient manages satisfactorily. Much of the time, however, failure to consider the family, community, and cultural context of illness blocks the physician from being effective with the patient. If we believe that individual, family, and societal influences are as important in producing illness as are microbes and disturbed biochemistry and genes, we have begun a revolution in medical thinking (4).

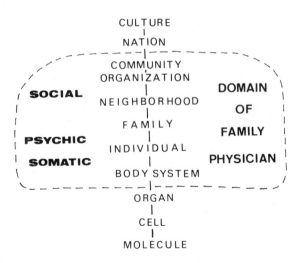

FIGURE 1.2. Systems hierarchy.

The History of Family Medicine/Practice

As medicine became more centralized in tertiary care teaching hospitals in the 1950s and 60s, it isolated itself from the community and public opinion. Hospitals, which have always been frightening places, became more confusing with the addition of new technology and many more personnel. Patients were generally treated paternalistically, having little or no say in their treatment. Families were mostly ignored, perceived as irritants or obstacles to be avoided or surmounted, rarely as allies in the healing process.

As the level of public sophistication about medical matters increased through media coverage and education, patients began expressing frustration with the insensitive, depersonalized approach of modern medicine. Women's groups and the consumer movement stepped up their criticisms. Ivan Illich summarized society's disillusionment in *Medical Nemesis:* "The medical establishment has become a major threat to health" (26). Iatrogenesis, illness arising from medical attention itself, was blamed for about 25% of hospital admissions. Physicians were accused of overmedicating patients, doing unnecessary surgery, and relying on technology to the exclusion of human interaction. In the 1960s, physicians were not readily available to the poor, the old, and those in rural areas. Although access to care has since improved greatly for most North Americans, other issues still persist—the greatly increased cost of health care, and the disproportionate amounts spent on some types of health care (e.g., coronary artery bypass).

Some medical leaders were also uncomfortable with such practices as referring to a patient as "the gallbladder in bed 3," and they shared the public concerns about the directions in which medicine was heading. In 1966 three "blue ribbon commission" reports appeared—the Millis Report (from the Citizens' Commission on Graduate Medical Education), the Folsom Report (from Health Services), and the Willard Report (from the Ad Hoc Committee on Education for Family Practice, from the AMA's Council on Medical Education) (27). All three pointed out the sharp reduction in the ratio of primary care physicians to secondary and tertiary care physicians in the United States, and the geographic maldistribution of physicians, with few doctors available in rural areas. They recommended that scientific medicine be combined with humanistic care of the whole patient in the context of his/her family.

These reports further recommended that a new specialty be established for family-oriented primary care, and in 1969 family medicine became the 21st specialty. In 1970 five family practice residency training programs were operating; in 1978 there were 348. This new specialty was designed to correct the results of an overreaction to the Flexner Report and the subsequent proliferation of medical technology. The patient was to be an equal partner in his/her own care, which was to be decentralized and to involve the patient's home environment.

The family physician's role is a bit paradoxical, in that he/she specializes in being a generalist. In a world moving toward ever narrower specialization (knowing more and more about less and less), the family physician is in some ways atavistic—a throwback to a former era. Because of the immense amount of cumulative medical knowledge, being a good generalist is an intellectually demanding, as well as a satisfying endeavor (28).

Another role the family physician has assumed is that of advocate for the patient in the complex medical system, mediating the care process in the outpatient and inpatient arenas of medicine—the tests and procedures, consultations and referrals to other specialists. This role has been referred to as gatekeeping, and is thought to be a crucial one in controlling the costs of care while preserving the quality of care. The modern physician has also assumed a central role in educating patients about their illnesses and about maintaining and enhancing their health. The shift toward more personalized care and attention to the consumer's outlook has led physicians to become more aware of how much patients' life circumstances influence the development and maintenance of symptoms and illness.

Most physicians become aware that families affect what they see people for in their offices. Since the family physician sees all age groups, he/she eventually notices that several family members get sick during a short time period, then no one from the family comes in for a while, and that this waxing and waning of symptoms correlates with rising and falling stress from outside and within the family. Symptoms reported by patients often do not match the diseases and syndromes learned in medical school. To understand what is going on, the family and community factors are the missing links.

Family practice has also revised the traditional paternalistic doctor–patient relationship. It is difficult for a family physician to act as the patient's ally while simultaneously maintaining a posture of father/priest/ M.D.eity. For the patient to be more in control of his/her illness, health, and life-style, a more egalitarian relationship is necessary, with the physician functioning as an expert adviser and coach, rather than a pompous pronouncer and dictator. In addition to the skills for taking charge of a very sick, helpless hospitalized patient, which medical students learn in most of their training, the physician needs to learn skills for negotiating and for empathizing nonjudgmentally, to allow patients to take responsibility for themselves and change their behavior.

Family medicine/practice emphasizes learning from illness, making new choices to produce growth, and becoming responsible in a more mature way (physician, patient, and family). The Chinese written character for crisis has two meanings: danger and opportunity. Good clinicians learn to foster learning and growth from crisis situations, a process Satir has described as the most valid function for the helping professions (29). Medicine may be incorporating this value into the biopsychosocial model proposed by Engel (3). Another whole discipline has been built on the premise that change can be promoted in time of crisis. The discipline is family therapy, and it has much to offer medicine in terms of understanding patients and families.

The History of Family Therapy

Like most of medicine, psychiatry has seen the individual as more or less isolated. Mental illness has been thought to be within the individual, albeit influenced by upbringing, especially early childhood experiences. In the 1950s Bateson and coworkers noticed that young schizophrenics often got better in the hospital, but within a week after returning to their families, they were again floridly psychotic (30). They observed that parents of schizophrenics often communicated in very rigid confused ways, verbally requesting the child to do one thing and nonverbally contradicting the verbal request or requesting something else. The child was in a "double bind"—damned if he did, and damned if he didn't. Another example of a double bind would be the requests, "Be spontaneous" and "Dominate me." Both contain a logical contradiction. If the person obeys, he/she is not being either spontaneous or dominant.

Families with schizophrenic members also displayed a great fearfulness about people outside the family, and a sense that their feelings were not

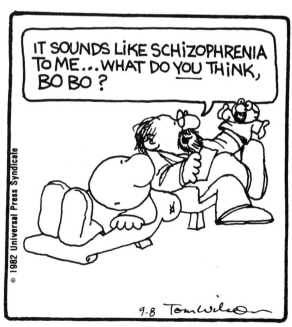

ZIGGY, by Tom Wilson. Copyright 1982, Universal Press Syndicate. Reprinted with permission. All rights reserved.

real or did not belong to them. Bowen interpreted these characteristics as reflections of emotional overinvolvement between family members (31). In many families, excessive emotional intensity exists between spouses, and between parents and children, because the individuals have poor differentiation of self-identity. All family members hold the family as a whole in low esteem. In such families, emotions are shared so pervasively that the origin of a feeling is unclear, and everyone feels a lack of ownership of feelings and an inability to control them. Families with members who are predisposed to schizophrenia (perhaps genetically, biochemically) and whose family dynamics resemble the above patterns, will be likely to produce one or more schizophrenic members. How does this come about?

Working with Bateson's group, Satir described communication styles that facilitated family functioning or family dysfunction (32). With congruent communication, verbal and nonverbal messages match, so that the overall message transmitted is a clear one. For example, the statement, "I like what you're doing," accompanied by a smile, is a congruent communication. In contrast, incongruent communication consists of mixed messages, such as "Don't do that," said with a smile to the 2-year-old recipient of the message.

The receiver of an incongruent message is confused about the true meaning of the communication, and has difficulty knowing how to respond to it. Much of the time, children and adults choose to respond to the nonverbal message, knowing from experience that it is more likely to be genuine than the verbal message. When the receiver responds to the non-verbal message, he/she often meets with a hostile or confused response from the original sender, because the sender may have been unaware of his/her own ambivalence and not in touch with the feeling that was tied to the nonverbal message.

In families with schizophrenic members, communication is quite in-

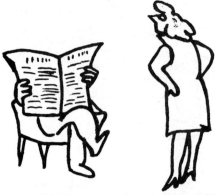

"I know you're listening—your knuckles are turning white."

congrent, with considerable confusion, especially when stress increases. If a schizophrenic member improves or gets well, the family tends to produce another symptomatic member (not necessarily schizophrenic). It is as if these families need someone to act crazy or be sick to keep the family in balance. From these observations researchers and clinicians derived the idea of "family homeostasis," similar to physiologic homeostasis (33). In one family, for example, the parents only began to complain about their son's crazy behavior, after years of psychotic symptoms, when he started roaming the streets at night. Previously he had been sleeping between the parents in bed, protecting them from facing touchy issues in their relationship as a couple.

Satir described four typical incongruent stances people use when their self-esteem is low or is threatened (32):

- *blaming* ("It's your fault. You always do it wrong. Do it my way.");
- *placating* ("Sorry, it's all my fault. I just want you to be happy, dear.");
- *super-reasonable* (denial of emotions—"Just give me the facts. My wife is the problem—she's too emotional."); or
- *irrelevant* (distracting or avoiding)
  - joking ("Death is just Nature's way of telling you to slow down.");
  - changing the subject ("That reminds me of the time Aunt Bess choked on a fish bone.");
  - leaving ("I'm going out for a walk.").

These stances are normal, though counterproductive, responses to stress and anxiety about feeling threatened. Blaming discounts the other person's feelings and evokes anger, and it covers up feelings of guilt or helplessness. Placating often covers feelings of repressed anger, as well as guilt; it evokes more abuse and disgust in the other person. A superreasonable person discounts all feelings, his/her own and those of others. Most physicians use the protection of hyperrationality for getting into and surviving medical school. The irrelevant stance indicates an internal state of hopelessness, since it discounts not only feelings, but also the rational context of the interaction. Most people are expert at one of the above stances, and well-versed in two of the others.

Incongruent communication stems from low self-esteem, originating in childhood (32). Parents with low self-esteem cannot express themselves honestly. They encircle the child with unspoken rules that prevent natural self-expression. Spontaneous acts are labeled as bad, and the child begins to feel he/she is no good. Parents who are well-intentioned and want the best for their children simply pass on the rules by which they were raised. Thinking well of oneself and caring for oneself are usually discouraged, and worth is measured only in achievements or the ability to be nice or good (inhibiting any negative emotions, which are considered bad).

The parents transmit their negative thinking and feelings to the child, who in turn grows up and transmits negativity to a spouse and to his/her own children. Often one child is targeted as the bad one. This may be a child the parents fight over, as they try to avoid conflict between themselves by "triangling in" a third party. If the parents' self-esteem and individuation levels are very low, a triangulated child may become schizophrenic or chronically ill in some other way (31). Minuchin worked with families of children with severe asthma, labile diabetes, and anorexia nervosa, all of whom were overly close (enmeshed) (18). In these families conflict was denied, and normal parental conflict was avoided by detouring it through the symptomatic child. For example, a child with a physiologic predisposition to asthma began to wheeze when the family tension rose and the parents began to argue. One parent then focused on the child's symptoms and took him to the emergency room, pushing the parental disagreement into the background.

Family therapy with such pyschosomatogenic families resulted in symptomatic improvement in all cases. The asthmatic children stopped having frequent visits to the emergency room and frequent hospitalizations, returned to school, and were able to discontinue steroid medication. The diabetic children were brought under good control, and their hospitalizations were reduced from up to 12 per year to an average of less than 1 a year.

These families were particularly reluctant to recognize their role in the illnesses. Families tend to resist change, even when the proposed change involves the improvement of a loved one (34). Change carries considerable risk and often exacts a high cost as one considers departing from and losing the familiar in exchange for exploring the scary unknown of new behavior. To help people navigate the perilous rapids of change, it is logical to regard the family as the unit of care, because the rocks that jeopardize successful passage are the hard family issues that must be dealt with in order for change to be made.

Family Systems Theory

Systems theory provides a nonjudgmental, and therefore relatively nonthreatening, framework for understanding families and helping them change. The myth that any one person is the problem, or is to blame for a family's difficulties, can only be exploded from outside the family system. The family is an interactional unit in which each person's steps in the "family dance" are influenced by every other member. Each member does the best he/she knows to solve problems that arise. Even in extreme cases of abuse or addiction, all family members contribute to the situation. Paradoxically, however, though no one is to blame, each member can be helped to realize that he/she is responsible for his/her own behavior, and that all he/she has the power to change is his/her own behavior.

General systems theory posits that the world is made up of interlocking interactional units of different levels of complexity. Each unit has a boundary that is variably permeable, an internal system of communication, and a means of communicating with outside systems (Figure 1.2). Each unit is in a state of dynamic homeostasis, maintained by positive and negative feedback mechanisms, with a central locus of control. A system is healthy if communication is clear and well organized by the central control body, and if the unit adapts well to changes in the surrounding systems (environment).

A healthy cell, for example, has a single nucleus that communicates effectively with the cellular components and the surrounding cells. A cancer cell loses these attributes. Cancer cells do not maintain well-organized patterns, and they do not respond to the boundaries of surrounding healthy cells. In a healthy system, the function of the part is subservient to the flourishing of the whole; reciprocally, the enhancement of the whole benefits each of the parts. Cancer cells become a destructive, self-serving part of a whole that then dies prematurely.

Similarly, a healthy family maintains a clear boundary around it that is open to influences from outside, and the family members communicate effectively with each other and with the outside world. The parents are in control, with a degree of organization that has enough flexibility to allow family members to grow and adapt to life circumstances. Even in healthy families, homeostasis can be disturbed by illness, and illness may be a symptom of the balance having being disturbed by other influences.

Systems principles are already familiar to the physician in the area of physiology. The principles of the endocrine system, for example, can be applied to family situations. A family from the first author's practice illustrates the parallels. The clinician's knowledge of five concepts from endocrinology can be transferred to the family system (see Figure 1.3)*:

1. The whole system must be understood in order to understand disease in any single organ.
2. Maintaining homeostasis is essential for the survival of the system; it is maintained by complex positive and negative feedback mechanisms.
3. One must consider not only the organs themselves, but also the interaction between the organs and the hormones they secrete. The hormones both affect other parts of the endocrine system, and indicate how the system is functioning.
4. Changes may occur in areas remote from the primary focus of pathology; all organs in the system may be affected by a change in one of them.
5. The endocrine system is hierarchical, and its healthy functioning depends on good communication between its components, particularly effective control through the cortical–hypothalamic–pituitary axis.

---

*This section on systems theory is reproduced with the publisher's permission, with minor revision, from Chapter 1 of the book *Working with Families in Primary Care: A Systems Approach to Health and Illness*, J. Christie-Seely, author–editor. New York, Praeger, 1984.

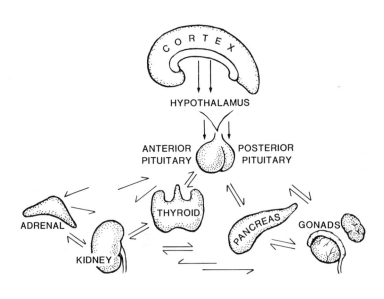

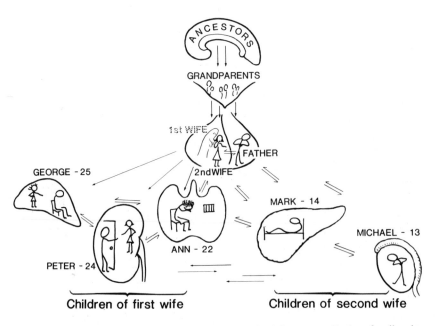

FIGURE 1.3.   Endocrine analogy of systems principles as applied to family situations.

Clinical Example #5: Systems Theory in Action

Using the biomedical model, the individual family members described below would have been seen, evaluated, and treated separately, with limited effectiveness.

Mr. B presented to his family physician with a bleeding peptic ulcer and hypertension. His poor compliance with antihypertensive medication later resulted in accelerated hypertension and renal failure. His second wife, the mother of his two youngest sons, Mark and Michael, visited the physician with frequent headaches. Two older sons, Peter and George, had unstable relationships with their girlfriends and returned home intermittently. First Mark, then Michael developed abdominal pain. The one daughter, Ann, had had several episodes of delinquency and suicide attempts. Both parents and two sons had thalassemia minor. At one point two family members developed giardiasis, a parasitic intestinal infection.

Using a family orientation, each family member is understood as part of a whole (Concept 1), as shown in Figure 1.3. Further important information came from family members once the family trusted the physician as a family confidante.

The father's first wife (portrayed as a ghost) died at the birth of Ann, the third child. The father had unresolved guilt over her death. The fact that she had hemorrhaged at home after the birth was a secret in the nuclear family, but the wife's family held Mr. B responsible for her death and ostracized him. Mr. B in turn ostracized his son, George, when he eventually married a girlfriend of whom the parents disapproved. The second wife had difficulty relating to the three older children. The family had a pattern of denial and avoidance of difficult topics, which was followed by physical illness or severed relationships. (The father said of George, "He is dead as far as I'm concerned.")

Homeostasis (Concept 2) was disturbed by Ann's developing sexuality and her resemblance to her dead mother, which increased her father's guilt and her stepmother's insecurity. The father's renal failure, which was never discussed, and the older boys leaving home further disrupted the equilibrium. Feedback mechanisms maintained the avoidance of conflict areas. Rather than openly face the father's illness and its implications, the family prompted the sons to come back home periodically, ostensibly as respite from the problems with their girlfriends, but functionally to take over the roles of fathering and breadwinning.

Ann similarly maintained the family denial by drawing the attention of the family and the medical profession to herself and away from the father's illness. Ann's feelings about her mother's death and her father's illness could not be dealt with directly without altering the family system in ways that were very threatening to the family.

To treat this family, a better understanding of family relationships was needed (Concept 3). The interaction of family members had to be observed, since the anxiety level was such that they were not objective observers of their own conflict avoidance. In an assessment interview with the whole family, the second wife's power became apparent. Normally reticent when seen alone, she was in complete charge of the assembled family. She answered all questions directed to her husband, and magnified his disability through overprotective concern. She showed obvious, but unspoken, jealousy of the dead wife and resentment of her stepdaughter, barely tolerating being in the same room with her. (When asked previously about their relationship, she said she got along very well with her stepdaughter.)

Diagnosis, treatment, and compliance were all improved by taking into account how individual symptoms or illness supported the disturbed family functioning. The purpose of intervention in such a family system is to induce a disequilibrium to break up the family complacency with the relatively stable dysfunction. The father's poor compliance had related to his guilt feelings for his first wife, and to his resisting the growing power of his second wife. The younger son's abdominal pains disappeared when their similarity to their father's ulcer symptoms was discussed.

The daughter, who was thought to be suffering from manic-depressive bipolar disorder or fugue disorder by a psychiatrist who evaluated her, was now seen to be behaving in fairly average ways considering the magnitude and nature of the family stresses. Helping the parents and the older sons with their difficulty leaving home led to improvements in the sons' relationships with their girlfriends.

In this family, unresolved grief and conflict over the death of the first wife reinforced preexisting obstacles to communication, with subsequent far-reaching effects on everyone in the family (Concept 4). As in most dysfunctional families, the couple relationship was the underlying problem. The husband buried his anger and guilt, abdicated his parental role, and undermined his wife's attempts to organize the family. The older sons tried to wrest control away from the wife on his behalf. The resulting unclear hierarchy and chaotic communication supported only poor functioning of the system, with the survival of the system and its members being jeopardized by the detrimental effects of chronic high anxiety levels (Concept 5).

Family therapy has added immeasurably to our understanding of families and how they are involved with individuals' health and illness. Family therapy offers the most effective therapeutic approach for some problems for which patients see doctors. It remains to be seen whether large numbers of physicians will adapt some of the skills of family therapists to help their patients, or whether most patients will continue to be referred to family therapists to receive this kind of help. It would be a major step forward if physicians could just learn to recognize families who might benefit from family therapy, and refer them skillfully.

Historical Perspective on the Family

The family continues to receive mixed reviews by scholars, politicians, and the media. It has long been the object of idealization, speculation, concern, and recrimination. On the one hand it is glorified: "The family, not the individual, is the real molecule of society, the key link in the social chain of being" (35). In other quarters the family is deprecated as "an institution for the systematic production of physical and mental illness in the members" (36).

Overall, the family is a lot like a sports coach or manager. It gets little credit for success when things are going well, but is blamed for failure when the going gets tough. Recent changes in families in many societies have prompted alarms that the family is no longer a stable institution, that it is no longer capable of performing its traditional function of socializing the next generation to preserve an orderly society. Some historic perspective may shed light on the degree to which these concerns are valid.

The mythical history of the family reads something like the following. In the good old days, the average family was one big happy family, with several generations living harmoniously under one roof for long periods of time—the cohabiting extended family. Some eight to ten children began to work at an early age to help the family subsist off the land by farming, gathering, hunting, and fishing. Marriage was for life, and divorce was almost unheard of, with divorcees being ostracized. People worked so hard to survive that they didn't develop many of the problems that plague us nowadays—e.g., anxiety and depression.

Juvenile delinquency didn't exist, since teenagers were busy working and didn't have any leisure time in which to misbehave. Welfare, social security, and nursing homes were unnecessary, because families took care of their own unfortunate and aging members, and when they couldn't, other more able families in the community did. Family members were born, lived, and died in the same community, rarely leaving even to visit other places, much less moving every 3 to 4 years like the modern ultramobile family. This idealized image is seen in the television families in "The Waltons" and "Little House on the Prairie."

What were things really like in the past? Recent studies of vital statistics records for the United States during the Colonial Period and the 1800s are revising our stereotyped ideas about the changing family. Although the divorce rate was low, husbands often abandoned their families (37). (The abandonment rate is now quite low, with wives leaving husbands more commonly.) Although first marriages were probably voluntarily discontinued less often in the past, there were several sources of involuntary discontinuation that may have almost equalized the overall endurance record for first marriages then and now. The mortality rate was substantially higher for young men, and considerably higher for young women, who often died from postpartum hemorrhage or infection. Remarriages of widows and widowers were very common in most genealogy records for the 19th century.

Because of these factors and the high infant mortality rate, the total number of children living in the average Colonial or 19th-century family at a given time appears to averaged only about three to four (37). Partly due to breast-feeding, the children were spread out over 15 to 20 years, so that at any given time the number of young children in the home was only about twice the two children now present in the average childbearing family.

How often did extended family members live with their adult relatives in the past? Apparently aging parents did live with adult children frequently, but due to earlier ages at death, these arrangements were seldom very prolonged. Many grown children moved away from their home community, often at the time of marriage, to establish independent lives and seek economic opportunities. American and Canadian families have apparently always been mobile and predominantly nuclear. Events like military induction and wars have contributed to the scattering of the younger generations.

What are the real differences in current family life? Many more women than ever before work outside the home and earn incomes comparable to (though still unfairly discrepant from) their husbands. The old stereotypical family consisting of a male breadwinner, a female homemaker, and several children accounted for only about 13% of all families in 1980 (38). The work load inside the home has been greatly reduced by the hundreds of laborsaving devices, leaving everyone who is not a workaholic with more leisure time than ever. Many families use this leisure time to strengthen their relationships, while many others mostly watch television. (Although the association between the rising divorce rate and the number of television sets in service is probably not a cause-and-effect relationship, it does raise the question of how family interactions are affected by members sitting transfixed, passively engaged with the television set instead of each other for hours at a time.)

Reflecting the increasing incidence of having children out of wedlock, and the divorce rate being approximately 50% for all first marriages after about 1980, an unparalleled number of homes contain only one full-time resident parent (16% of all families in 1980) (38). This is especially true for black families headed by unmarried women, although these numbers are somewhat misleading. Studies have found that there is usually a supportive male in the picture nearby, who is present in the home intermittently and functions in the roles of husband and father. True single-parent families are vulnerable to destabilization by illness or other adverse events, since they have less coping reserve than comparable two-parent families.

Because of the high divorce and remarriage rates, many households now contain "blended" families with children from two or more different marriages. These families have all the usual difficulties of first-time marriages, compounded by the dynamics of the rift between the biologic parents and the complexities of the step relationships. Some families handle the situation well, with both parents continuing to be involved with various joint custody arrangements. Other families continue to fight their battles for years through the children, from different headquarters.

Another real difference between families today and those of the past derives from the steady increase in life expectancy and the reduction in childbearing past the age of 35. The net result is that, if the offspring leave the home on schedule at age 18–20, and the marriage has survived, the couple faces the prospect of several more decades of living together, some 30 or more years on the average, unless one of the partners dies. This lengthy period together at the end of life is the major new development for the 20th-century Western family, and it presents difficult problems for many couples who discover they have little in common after the children are gone. The fact that marriages today can potentially last 50–70 years is an unparalleled experiment in togetherness, for which we are ill-prepared.

Because people live longer and can travel and communicate over long distances more easily now, more adults are in touch with their aging parents than at any time since the widespread increase in nuclear family mobility. Grandchildren and grandparents see and talk to each other more now while living far apart. This increased contact holds the potential for both favorable interaction and long-range conflict. Grandparents, especially grandmothers, are often extremely influential in matters of health and illness, even if living at great distance. It is wise to solicit the grandmother's opinion if she comes with a sick grandchild, or to inquire about the opinions of grandparents when seeing children with health problems.

Overall the family has undergone some significant changes in the last several decades. In the past it has always adapted flexibly to changes in society, modifying its primary functions or altering the ways in which it

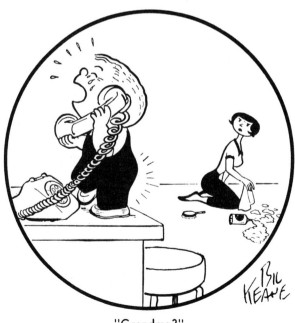

"Grandma?"

achieved them. Although the family as we have known it or have imagined it may be dying, the demise of the family itself has been greatly exaggerated.

What Makes a Family More or Less Healthy?

Family life is very important to almost everyone. According to a 1980 Harris survey, 96% of Americans listed having a "good family life" at the top of the list of goals they have for themselves. What is a "good family life?" What is a healthy family like, compared to an unhealthy family?

All happy families are alike;
every unhappy family is unhappy in its own way.—Tolstoy (39)
All happy families are more or less dissimilar;
all unhappy ones are more or less alike.—Nabokov (40)

Both of the above quotes are correct. Healthy families share some common traits and have some features that distinguish them from each other. Unhealthy families also share some common traits and have distinctive variations. Much of this book will discuss how to deal with unhealthy families. It is useful to keep in mind that all families have strengths, some more than others. To help an individual, it is as important to identify the strengths of a family as it is to detect its weaknesses.

Some of the people studying families in the past two decades have tried to identify how healthy families resembled each other, and how they were different from less functional families. One noted study found that no single characteristic clearly distinguished families that produced highly functioning offspring from those whose children had serious problems. Several features were shared by most of the healthy families, including a strong marital alliance that met the needs of both parents well, and effective communication of thoughts and feelings (41).

An interesting book on traits of a healthy family was based on a large survey of professionals who work with families regularly (42). The consensus opinion was that members of healthy families:

- communicate effectively, especially during regular shared meals;
- respect and support each other;
- respect others outside the family;
- trust each other;
- share time together with play and humor, balanced among family members;
- take responsibility for their actions;
- teach and learn morals that promote the common good and individual welfare;
- enjoy traditions (holiday gatherings, rituals, ceremonies);
- share a religious belief;
- respect each other's privacy;

- value service to others;
- admit to problems and seek help for them when necessary.

Many families do reasonably well without some of the things listed above, but the more of them missing from family life, the less likely it is that the family can perform its essential functions. For the family to meet the basic needs of its members and of society, it must:

1. Physically protect and sustain its members by providing shelter, safety, food, and clothing (not necessarily designer jeans).
2. Promote a sense of individuality or autonomy, so that each member can think and feel independently, when that is appropriate.
3. Promote a sense of connectedness, so that each member meets emotional needs for affection and intimacy appropriately, reproduces in a responsible way, and cooperates with others when indicated.
4. Foster a sense of competence and self-worth, so that each member feels good about him/herself and contributes productively to society.
5. Encourage each member to develop a sense of right and wrong and conform to the most basic values and rules of society (respect the rights of others).

The physician who approaches patients and families nonjudgmentally will facilitate self-acceptance, which is often a prerequisite for change. Emphasizing strengths promotes health and growth. Antonovsky showed that a sense of coherence (having a rightful place in a reasonably ordered world) correlated with health (43). Families with high rates of divorce, delinquency, and dysfunction also were shown by Hinkle and Wolff to have early disease, disability, and death (44). Members of illness-prone families generally have low self-esteem and are poorly individuated. (See Chapters 3, 7, and 9 for more on this topic.)

Summary

Medicine is slowly reawakening to the importance of family influences on health and illness. Public awareness has driven or kept pace with the emerging new disciplines of family medicine and family therapy. The family appears to be adapting effectively to changes in Western society and maintaining its viability as the fundamental unit of society. Because of the seriousness of the problems within many families and the dilemmas of society, individuals and families often become symptomatic and seek help from physicians. Sorting out and dealing with information from multiple systems levels is an exciting challenge for physicians of the future.

References

1. Carmichael LP, Carmichael L: The relational model in family practice. Marriage Fam Rev 1981;4:123.
2. Kuhn IS: The Structure of Scientific Revolutions, ed 2. Chicago, University of Chicago Press, 1970.

3. Engel GL: The need for a new medical model: A challenge for biomedicine. Science 1977;196:129.
4. McWhinney I: Family medicine as a science. J Fam Pract 1978;7:53.
5. Ransom DC: The rise of family medicine: new roles for behavioral sciences, in Cogswell BE, Sussman MB (eds): Family Medicine: A New Approach to Health Care. New York, Haworth Press, 1982, pp 31–72.
6. Glenn M: On Diagnosis: A Systemic Approach. New York, Brunner/Mazel, 1984.
7. McWhinney I: Beyond diagnosis: an approach to the integration of behavioral science and clinical medicine. N Engl J Med 1972;384:387.
8. Zola IK: Studying the decision to see a doctor. Adv Psychosom Med 1972;8:216.
9. Christie-Seely JE: Life stress and illness: A systems approach. Can Fam Physician 1983;29:533.
10. Kraus AS, Lillienfeld AM: Some epidemiological aspects of the high mortality rate in the young widowed group. J Chron Dis 1959;3:207.
11. Christie-Seely J, Guttman H: The relevance of the family to medical outcomes, in Christie-Seely J (ed): Working with the Family in Primary Care: A Systems Approach to Health and Illness. New York, Praeger Publishers, 1984, chap 9.
12. Balint M: The Doctor, His Patient, and the Illness. New York, International Universities Press, 1972.
13. Gore S: The effect of social support in moderating the health consequences of unemployment. J Health Soc Behav 1978;19:157.
14. Gerber I, Wiever A, Battin D, et al: Brief therapy to the aged bereaved, in Schoenberg B, Gerber I (eds): Bereavement: Its Psychosocial Aspects. New York, Columbia University Press, 1975.
15. Raphael, B: Preventive intervention with the recently bereaved. Arch Gen Psychiatry 1977;34:1950.
16. Christie-Seely J: Psychological problems of adults: "Individual problems," in Christie-Seely J (ed): Working with the Family in Primary Care: A Systems Approach to Health and Illness. New York, Praeger Publishers, 1984, chap 24.
17. Feldman LB: Depression and marital interaction. Fam Process 1976;14:389.
18. Minuchin S, Baker L, Rosman BL, et al: A conceptual model of psychosomatic illness in children: Family organization and family therapy. Arch Gen Psychiatry 1975;32:1031.
19. Minuchin S, Rosman BL, Baker L: Psychosomatic Families: Anorexia Nervosa in Context. Cambridge, MA, Harvard University Press, 1978.
20. Chambers WN, Reiser MF: Emotional stress in the precipitation of heart failure. Psychosom Med 1953;14:38.
21. Richardson HP: Patients Have Families. New York, Commonwealth Fund, 1945.
22. Flexner A: Medical Education in the United States and Canada: A Report to the Carnegie Foundation for the Advancement of Teaching. Boston, DB Updike, Merrymount Press, 1910.
23. Pearse I, Crocker L: The Peckham Experiment: A Study in the Living Structure of Society. London, Allen and Unwin, 1943.
24. Silver GA: Family Medical Care: A Design for Health. Cambridge, MA, Ballinger, 1974.

25. Brody H: The systems view of man: Implications for medicine, science and ethics. Perspect Biol Med 1973;17:71.
26. Illich I: Medical Nemesis. New York, Pantheon Books, 1976.
27. Cogswell BE: Family physician: A new role in process of development, in Cogswell BE, Sussman MB (eds): Family Medicine: A New Approach to Health Care. New York, Haworth Press, 1982, pp 1–30.
28. Stephens GG: The Intellectual Basis of Family Practice. Tucson, AZ, Winter Publishing, 1982.
29. Satir V. Conjoint Family Therapy: A Guide to Theory and Technique. Palo Alto, CA, Science and Behavior Books, 1964.
30. Bateson G, Jackson D, Haley J, Weakland J: Toward a theory of schizophrenia. Behav Sci 1956;1:251.
31. Bowen M. Family Therapy in Clinical Practice. New York, Jason Aronson, 1978.
32. Satir V. Peoplemaking. Palo Alto, CA, Science and Behavior Books, 1972.
33. Jackson DD: The question of family homeostasis. Psychiatr Q 1957;31(suppl):79.
34. Hoffman L. Foundations of Family Therapy: A Conceptual Framework for Systems Change. New York, Basic Books, 1972.
35. Nisbet R. Twilight of authority, in Howard J (ed): Families. New York, Simon and Schuster, 1978, p 11.
36. Montagu A: in Howard J (ed): Families. New York, Simon and Schuster, 1978, p 63.
37. Seward RR: The American Family: A Demographic History. Beverly Hills, CA, Sage Publications, 1978.
38. Households and families by type: March 1980. Fam Econ Rev 16 (Winter) 82-040. [Listed in Index to Government Periodicals, 1982.]
39. Tolstoy LN: Anna Karenina. New York, Dodd, Meade & Co., 1966, part 1, chap 1.
40. Nabokov V: Ada (or Ardor: A Family Chronicle). New York, McGraw-Hill, 1969.
41. Lewis JM, Beavers WR, Gossett JT, Phillips VA: No Single Thread: Psychological Health in Family Systems. New York, Brunner/Mazel, 1976.
42. Curran D: Traits of a Healthy Family. Minneapolis, Winston Press, 1983.
43. Antonovsky A: Health, Stress and Coping. San Francisco, Jossey-Bass, 1979.
44. Hinkle LE, Wolff HG: Ecological investigation of the relationship between illness, life experience, and the social environment. Ann Intern Med 1958;49:1373.

CHAPTER 2

A Systems View of the Clinical Relationship

Howard F. Stein

What Is a Systemic View?

The clinical relationship is the foundation of all clinical action. Technical proficiency and communication skills are necessary but not sufficient components of this relationship. In this chapter, various *systemic features of the clinical relationship* are explored. From a systemic view actions are influenced by a wide range of ongoing processes. "Systemic features" refer to the nature of the larger network of relationships and meanings that influence clinical assessment, diagnosis, and treatment. Facets of this larger system include the physician's own established unconscious and conscious behavioral patterns, the physician–patient interaction, the doctor–patient–family relationship, the interplay of members of the health care team, and the impact of perceptions of time and business issues upon patient care. This systemic approach reveals the world of clinical reality to be far more complex than is commonly believed. The added complexity may often constrain clinical decision making and impede the clinician's wishes to heal with standard simplified interventions. On the other hand, the physician who explores the meanings and relationships in this system will discover new intervention opportunities. This chapter describes some of the many systems that enter into all aspects of the physician–patient relationship.

This chapter identifies and discusses three categories of influences upon the clinical relationship: (a) *persons* (e.g., the physician, the patient, members of the physician's and patient's families of origin and current families, medical and administrative members of the health care team); (b) *institutions, occasions,* and *places* that affect the clinical relationship (e.g., the clinic, the hospital, insurance companies, the patient's home, staff meetings, case conferences, local and national government); and (c) *issues* that impinge upon the clinical relationship (e.g., language and metaphor, time, clinical process, content and outcome, levels of analysis of clinical problems, participants' interpretations of the nature and meaning of the illness episode, public accountability, cost containment, cultural ethos, countertransference, etc.) (see Figure 2.1). Of course, all three categories are facets of the same clinical relationship, and no institutions, occasions, places, and issues occur apart from the people who constitute them.

With regard to the dimensions of the clinical relationship, what has been said well elsewhere is not recounted here. Several original references contain much excellent information about the doctor–patient relationship. Balint (1) and Devereux (2) explored the psychodynamic dimension of medical practice for the practitioner as well as the patient. Szasz and Hollender (3) described the parent–child, parent–adolescent, and adult–adult styles of interaction. Froelich and Bishop (4) explained basic clinical communication skills and how to use them. Kleinman (5) carefully described the interplay between the physician's biomedical "explanatory model" and the patient's own cultural "explanatory model" in clinical transactions. Katz (6) and Stein (7,8) discussed psychodynamic and contextual issues in medical practice. Doherty and Baird (9) applied principles of family dynamics and family therapy to the practice of primary care medicine.

The goal of this chapter is to explore how a systemic approach can help the physician be a better clinician, diagnostician, and manager, in part by encouraging the physician to be more accepting of limits set by the situation upon intervention options. Paying close attention to the interplay of *multiple* relationship systems in medicine may allow the clinician to better understand what is taking place in the family with which he/she is working. The patient and family are no more an isolated unit than is the cell. To understand what is happening with a cell, one must not only know a lot about organelles, but also much about the cell's environment.

Consider the following case vignette. Nancy N is a 36-year-old midwestern American divorcee with two teenage children. She supports her family by working as an enterprising business executive. She prides herself on her self-reliance and self-sufficiency. Recently undergoing a hysterectomy, she amazed physicians and hospital staff alike with her strength and resilience; she withstood considerable pain without calling for medication. She cut her expected 6 to 8 weeks' recovery time in half. She was eager to return to work, worried that responsibilities would pile up, and concerned that money to run the household would be depleted.

Her parents, retired out of state, insisted on coming to spend several weeks with her to help her recuperate from surgery. Arriving a week prior to surgery, they stayed until about a week afterward. The day before their arrival, she thoroughly cleaned the house for fear her mother would criticize her housekeeping ("Mother would be sure to notice crumbs or dirt under the toaster and proceed to clean the house if I didn't."). While her parents were in her home, she was cheerful, talkative, and active around the house. Although her parents had come to take care of her, she refused to allow them to do so, but instead took care of herself *and* them. She later explained: "I don't act sick so they won't worry." They left satisfied that she was recovering well.

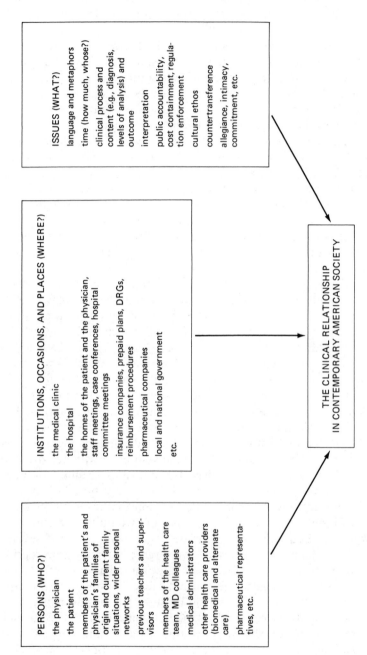

FIGURE 2.1.   Schematic of system components of the clinical relationship.

Only after her parents had gone did she allow herself to feel and act sick at home (i.e., take on the sick role). She looked tired and pale. Although still surprisingly energetic, she did not keep going on tirelessly for hours as she had when her parents were there. She allowed herself to rest and sleep only when she had reclaimed her home and her privacy. From the perspective of clinic and hospital visits, most physicians would regard this woman as a good if not ideal patient. Becoming familiar with her world through interviewing and observing her at home shed a far different light on her illness behavior.

Peeling the Onion in Clinical Practice

Many medical problems resemble the metaphorical "onion." When scrutinized closely they shed layer after layer, as in the preceding case. This does not mean that the outer layers are less vivid, urgent, and real than the deeper, more obscure ones. Rather, it means that the outer level is not the whole story, and that the "onion" problem will not be entirely resolved by attending solely to the outer level. At times a strictly biomedical viewpoint may oversimplify and mislead the direction of our assessment and care. At times we may need to "peel the onion" to manage symptoms unresponsive to a reductionistic view of the presenting illness (e.g., "the gallbladder in room 242").

Consider the following scenario. A physician sees a 6-month-old undernourished male "preemie" brought to the emergency room by a babysitter. The baby has gained a meager 10 pounds. During subsequent hospitalization, within 1 week the baby gains 1.7 pounds. The mother, 18 years old, now divorced, rarely visits her infant in the hospital, and has little eye contact with him when she does visit. We learn that the mother had herself been abandoned when she was 5 months old. How do these layers of available information influence the treatment plan for this malnourished child? Can the child alone remain the focus of treatment? How can the physician take into account important people in the patient's natural environment, such as the babysitter?

We must be able to accurately describe the patient's life situation before we can propose changes in that situation. The danger with any model is that the viewer sees reality only through the lens of the model, and thereby only takes note of what the model instructs him/her to focus on. Trying to be precise without tolerating reasonable uncertainty shapes one's observations to fit preexisting dogma. Heavily biased observation produces neither good science nor good medicine (10–12). On the other hand, a naturalistic approach of listening and observing with minimal preconceptions about what constitutes the patient's significant context can help minimize such distortion. This approach facilitates clinical assessment, communication, and intervention alike.

For example, several health professionals tried to explain the problem of premature ventricular contractions to family members of a midwestern farmer whose scheduled surgery had been abruptly postponed. Biomedical drawings and technical language failed to help them understand what was going on. Finally, an old general practitioner said simply that the farmer's heart "was shimmying like the front end of a Chevy pickup," and they were completely satisfied. This physician conveyed *his* (biomedical) world to the family of the patient in language that made sense to them and that thereby diminished their anxiety. The patient and family who feel they and their world are taken seriously are more likely to try to take the physician and the physician's world more seriously than if no such bridge is made. The physician needs to take the first step to find a common language that physician, patient, and family can understand and accept.

In America, many patients and their families expect that if they present their symptom(s) to the doctor, after a certain amount of verbal and physical examination and laboratory tests, the doctor will be able to "fix it." One thus hands one's body over to the physician to work on just as one turns over one's faulty car to the automobile mechanic. Many physicians approach medical practice with similar attitudes and expectations. Often this approach works because it fits the patient's, family's, and physician's model and expectation of outcome (e.g., symptom relief or reassurance that no major disease process is taking place).

The physician must pay attention to the potential meaning and function that patients and families may attach to symptoms and diseases. Multiple layers of problems may lurk beneath the presenting and official family symptom(s) and diagnosis. Somatic symptoms often serve as a family myth that prevents deeper, more painful feelings from surfacing (13).

Clinical Example #1

A mother in her late 20s was referred by her internist to a family therapist to deal with her persistent fears that her 10-year-old son was becoming schizophrenic. The mother became hyperattentive to the boy's every move. A quiet, somewhat shy boy, he was acting normally for his age, yet his mother was convinced that many of his behaviors signaled schizophrenia. In therapy, her preoccupation with the 10-year-old came to be understood as a way of distracting the family's attention away from their concerns about their 8-year-old diabetic girl. By obsessing about the son's supposed withdrawal, they were able to avert and deny their fear of their daughter's death.

The diabetes in turn served as a safety valve for a marriage rife with simmering conflict. Anxiety about the marital friction was detoured into a preoccupation with the daughter's brittleness. It was her death—not the threat of the end of the marriage and family—that then occupied everyone's attention. Further along, the therapist uncovered yet another family secret: the husband's long-standing drinking (approximately 12 beers per day, every day of the year). The wife had kept this problem hidden lest the family be shamed by the knowledge becoming public. As the marital strife and the husband's alcoholism were discussed, the woman and therapist discovered yet another layer of the onion of unresolved problems: the patient and her mother were both chronically anxious. Their anxiety stemmed from their own incomplete separation from one another, and was expressed in their respective marital problems. As the woman began to examine issues that derived their toxicity from her family of origin, she saw her current family issues as less mysterious and ominous and began to deal with them more realistically.

Clinical Example #2*

Jenny Kraft is a 17-year-old caucasian midwestern American teenager who developed anorexia nervosa 4 years ago. Her father and stepmother brought her to their family physician when she had lost considerable weight from not eating. The family physician requested consultation and saw the patient and family together with the consultant therapist during her hospitalization and during subsequent individual and family sessions. Precisely how family issues were involved in the etiology and persistence of the anorexia emerged only after many weeks, as the practitioners became familiar with family patterns of communication: e.g., the stepmother would insist on obtaining Jenny's opinion about some subject and then castigate if not slap her for being "wrong." Jenny threw away her birth control pills for fear that her stepmother would surmise she was having intercourse if she found out Jenny was taking them. One factor in particular suggested that the problem lay in the whole family, not just in Jenny, the identified patient. Both physician and consultant felt overwhelmed and confused when meeting with the family. This response generally reflects a profound problem of unclear boundaries in the family—a lack of definition of individual identity and generational separation.

Jenny was the eldest female sibling in a reconstituted family of 8 children. Her father was a farmer and cattle rancher who spent most of his time tending his fields and cattle. For him work was his all-male refuge from family. Her stepmother was a conscientious woman in her 40s who cared for home and children, and who felt overwhelmed by domestic responsibility. Husband and wife interacted little directly, and mostly over various conflicts with the children. The marital role was not only subordinate to the parental role, it was virtually nonexistent.

Individual and family therapy revealed that Jenny had begun to use self-starvation as a desperate attempt to establish distinct personal boundaries, especially from her stepmother, to whom Jenny felt very close but whom she was never able to please. She called her stepmother "Mom" affectionately, and regarded her as her mother. She was also unconsciously using her symptoms to stave off sexual development, for to become a woman was to be trapped. Jenny's natural mother had abandoned her when Jenny was 8. Her stepmother subsequently enlisted her to be a junior mother in the joint family, consuming most of Jenny's time and energy outside school. Her father expected her to bring home perfect grades, and both parents closely supervised such high school activities as gymnastics and cheerleading. Her stepmother followed her every move and demanded

---

*Originally presented in Stein HF: Values and family medicine. In Schwartzman J (ed): Families and Other Systems. New York, Guilford Press, 1985, pp. 236–239.

constant reports from her. Her parents' approval was very important to Jenny. She tried hard to live up to their exacting expectations.

The age of 17 was significant for Jenny's stepmother, for it was at 17 that *she* had left her parental home, married, begun bearing children, and shouldered enormous responsibilities in a small Oklahoma farm community. Jenny, who had been flirting on and off with marriage, felt compelled to get married that year, but was simultaneously repelled by the idea. She vacillated between wanting to be a dutiful daughter and wanting to make a complete break with her family. The prospect of marriage was the main potential vehicle for escaping (as it had been for her stepmother). In interactions with her boyfriend and her parents, she likewise alternated between clinging and fleeing.

Six months into therapy, Jenny ran away from home with her boyfriend, and her parents initiated a desperate state-wide search for her. She returned on her own choice within 2 days, having escaped detection, remorseful for having caused her family so much grief. In a subsequent family therapy session, the atmosphere was grave. The father was silent and sullen, the stepmother fought tears and anger. Finally, the stepmother said sobbing, but with resolve in her voice: "I wish to God I had the courage to run away." This was a breakthrough in the treatment. The stepmother made no immediate connection between her own feelings of imprisonment, her inability to do anything except continue to bear the family's burdens in silence, her own desire to run away, and her stepdaughter's acting out of her forbidden wish. Gradually, however, the stepmother came to understand that the more she could confidently stand up to her husband with her own principles, needs, expectations, and limits, the less she would feel the panicky need to flee from an impossible situation, and the less she would covertly encourage her stepdaughter to do (in her behalf) what she could not do herself.

In the next family session, the stepmother was openly angry about having allowed her fears of being alone, abandoned, helpless, and the like to dominate her actions and compel her to hold the family together. She permitted herself to set some limits on others' demands. On previous occasions, she had let her appearance go. On this day she had fixed her hair nicely, wore a stunning outfit, and smiled for the first time since the initial meeting. She gradually discovered that she needed her depression less as an escape from an unbearable reality that she had helped to fashion (and as punishment for the wish to escape). Over time she dealt with her current reality less masochistically. For instance, she gave herself permission to let the roof keep leaking until her husband made time to repair it, rather than assuming responsibility for fixing it herself. Jenny's anorexia nervosa and vacillation between flight and clinging likewise began to resolve. This was possible only after we had located her personal problems within the multiple contexts of individual development, family history, current family relationships, and the significance of work within the family.

Over time in clinical relationships layers of meaning may gradually unfold like those above. The physician who can disregard the myth that medical knowledge must be complete after a few minutes with the patient or after a few tests is in a better position to treat the patient and/or family as they are rather than as he/she would like them to be. When appropriate, the physician who patiently gathers information over several visits can make an effective referral, one that is not superficial—a referral that conveys thoroughness rather than riddance. The busy physician who does not wish to work with such complicated patients and families can at least do a thorough initial assessment that does not seriously understate the complexity of the problem.

Finally, the image of the onion is a useful metaphor for approaching cases. Each physician can decide how much of each particular onion he/she wants to peel, and how much to delegate to another clinician. As with peeling a real onion, the clinician may find it more and more difficult to face the increasing intensity of the inner layers. Sharing or referring difficult cases is analogous to improving the ventilation while peeling an onion—the clinician's vision stays clear enough to do a good job.

Vulnerabilities in the Clinical Relationship

Physicians often measure their professional and personal competence exclusively by their ability to change or cure their patients. Thus the doctor invests the patient with the power to determine the doctor's own self-worth—a burden for patient and doctor alike. When a patient relapses or dies, when a physician cannot reverse a chronic or life-threatening condition, the doctor's feelings of guilt and self-recrimination can become remorseless and dangerous to the doctor's own health.

(from a practicing family physician in his mid-50s):Sometimes I feel old. I've got a patient I've seen for twenty years. He's in the ICU with congestive heart failure. I think we're going to lose him. I've gone down the road with him for so many different things over the years; each time I was able to do something for him, to bring him back to normal functioning. It was a great feeling to see him walk out of the hospital. I got to know his whole family. I knew I was doing some good. But maybe I'm losing my touch, or the magic isn't what it used to be. You get to a point with a patient when you can't do it any more, and you remember what you used to be able to do. [I interjected: "Do you feel guilty and like a failure at times like these?"] You sure do. You say to yourself: "You turned things around before, how come you can't now?" You don't want to let your patients down, you don't want to stand by helplessly, yet everybody's got to die sometime.

It is as important for physicians to know strategically when to "let go" of their patients—to relinquish a struggle for control, to recognize the doctor's limitations and the patient's responsibility—as it is to know when to take command of the situation. The ability to mourn with and for one's patients is an underrated clinical skill; it is as important as is the ability to cure and save.

The Systemic View as Expansion of the Biomedical View

While the focus of attention is current family and family-derived forces, a wide range of factors need to be taken into account as systems components during assessment, history taking, therapeutic intervention, and outcome determination. Such factors include: the intrapsychic world of the patient; the emotional system of the family; relationships at work; one's personal network of friends, neighborhood, church, and voluntary organizations; and the medical and administrative personnel in the health care system, including the family physician (14–17). Information about these spheres is often indispensable to obtaining a more complete clinical picture of the persistence, if not also the etiology, of the symptom pattern (18,19).

Sometimes the physician and the health care system become adopted as a patient's quasi-family. In 1969 Earley and von Mering wrote about many Americans "growing old the outpatient way" (20) and using clinic and hospital visits as more social than medical occasions. Everyone involved in medicine knows the extent to which the emergency room and hospital have been used (many say, abused) as a refuge and sanctuary from the demands and conflicts of family and work. On the one hand the medical model expects us to cure people so that they will not have to come back for further treatment, while, on the other, for some patients the goal is to maintain the human relationship at all costs. At times the intense attachment is not so much to an individual practitioner as it is to an institution and what it represents to the patient (21).

Influences upon the Clinical Relationship

If physicians have an especially keen sense of responsibility toward their patients, they may have problems with control issues (e.g., patient compliance). For these doctors, work with many patients often becomes exasperating. They unwittingly find themselves in the position of trying to please their professional parents (faculty) through successfully controlling patient behavior. Or they may repeat patterns from their family of origin (e.g., being overly apologetic with certain patients, lecturing some, being angry at others). Patterns internalized from one's family of origin can powerfully influence the clinical relationship and patient care in ways the clinician is often unaware of (22).

Clinical Example #3*

A second-year Family Medicine resident requested consultation concerning a 40-year-old alcoholic male. The precipitating event for his most recent alcoholic binge (the first in 8 months) was a truck accident. He wrecked the truck, but was not fired by his employer. Instead, the patient left the job convinced that he was a failure. In a patterned sequence he tried to do something good, became depressed, consumed alcohol, and attempted or contemplated suicide.

As the resident discussed the case with her consultant, the initial focus was on patient history, a review of management history, and similar patient-centered issues. The resident then somewhat sarcastically brought up her own "mothering tendencies." When asked to continue, she said that she found herself in frustrating situations like this with other men whom she had tried to help. In fact, this patient reminded her of one of her four younger brothers. She characterized this eldest brother as unreliable, as one who always gets himself in trouble and needs to be rescued; her own role had been to rescue him.

Both in her family situation and in her clinical situation, the resident felt called upon to provide a remedy, to save a victim in distress. Only by taking care of them could she feel good about herself. Her mother had experienced numerous illness episodes when the resident was young, and had asked her daughter to take full responsibility for the care of the three brothers. The resident had felt responsible to her mother for the brother's behavior and felt guilty when she could not help her brother.

Just as her patient felt himself to be a failure, the resident's inability to control him or to help him made her likewise feel a failure. She became both angry with him and depressed about herself. With this discovery and understanding of her own tendencies, she was able to delineate more clearly the boundary between her family of origin and her current clinical relationship. Over time, with this patient and others, she felt less compelled to repeat her mothering tendencies, and became more realistic about how responsible to feel for her patients' welfare, actions, and outcome.

Far more people, institutions, and issues impinge on the apparent confidentiality of the clinical relationship than meets the eye. Consider, for instance, the simple act of writing a prescription for the patient, a matter seemingly influenced only by the physician's scientific knowledge as it is applied to the best interests of the patient. Yet how a given doctor prescribes medication may be influenced by the clinical habits and preferences of clinical teachers with whom he/she spent much time during medical training (6). That is, the supposedly scientific selection of the drug of choice for a patient may be silently mediated by a previous authority figure whose answers during one's training days still influence the former trainee's behavior.

---

*Originally presented in Stein HF: The Psychodynamics of Medical Practice: Unconscious Factors in Patient Care. Berkeley, University of California Press, 1985, pp 31–35.

Moreover, physicians are constantly subjected to the hidden persuaders of medical advertising, which tries to influence one's clinical judgment using popular cultural symbols. Pharmaceutical representatives frequently visit the training and practicing sites of physicians and provide free samples of medicine, various "freebies" (calendars, calipers, pens), and meals.They may even become personal friends of physicians. Thus the prescribing of medication for patient and family may be complicated by the participation of other relationships the doctor has that may influence clinical decision making.

Clinical consensus achieved in a group is sometimes useful, but can lead the clinician astray. One may be led to treat the patient for what has been selectively interpreted through projection by the group onto the patient (1,7,8). The group may unwittingly displace its own biases or problems onto the patient. When groups of health personnel gather to discuss patient care, more or less exclusive attention to biomedical diagnostic and management issues may be used defensively to stereotype patients who are poor, elderly, or culturally divergent. Indeed, powerful group fantasies can distort diagnosis and treatment to prove their truth (23).

Clinical Example #4

At a joint Family Medicine/Pastoral Counselor case conference the group quickly presumed that the sudden illness of an 85-year-old woman was a typical decline of mental and physical functions. For over an hour general prejudice toward the aged ("They're all alike") was expressed until one member jolted the team back to reality by reiterating the *acute* onset of the patient's paranoid symptoms. Her actual situation had not been addressed, but rather the elderly stereotype, thus obscuring the pertinent clinical data. The group's diagnostic pessimism and fatalism abated as the fantasy about the patient was dispelled and the actual facts analyzed. It subsequently turned out that the pastor's regular visits to the patient's home, together with medical management, restored this woman to her normal state of health and independence.

Hospital and Home Visits: Where to See the Family?

The primary care physician often identifies situations in which the family might be usefully convened (24). A request to bring the family together in the clinic may be declined, however, if it is considered inconvenient or unnecessary by some of the family's members. The physician, for instance, might diagnose a patient's anorexia nervosa as a family problem, while the parents may well regard it exclusively as "our daughter's eating problem." When a patient is hospitalized, however, many families congregate around the bedside of their sick member. Hospitalization is an opportune time for the observant physician to meet with the family partly on the family's terms. The physician must keep in mind, however, that many families view the hospital more as a place to die than a place to be cured. Hospitalization frequently constitutes a crisis. In a crisis the family's receptivity to outside assistance and willingness to consider change may be either heightened or diminished, depending on their flexibility. If the physician approaches the family, his/her assistance is most often welcomed. The astute physician can likewise invite hospital nurses to observe and report family interactions when appropriate and not intrusive.

The logic that suggests that the physician try to meet with the family in the hospital (to obtain as well as to convey information) also commends the use of the well-timed "home visit." A single home visit may be worth many office visits. From such a visit the family may derive deep feelings of trust, commitment, and being taken seriously by the clinician. Home visits are especially useful when: (a) a number of office approaches (including medication changes and in-clinic family consultations) have failed to effect a change; (b) the biomedical assessment is clear-cut and complete but the physician senses that something else is exacerbating or prolonging the symptoms; or (c) the problem appears to be a multiperson problem, and the physician wants to directly assess the patient's natural context that sustains that problem (25).

In both the hospital family visit and home visit the physician may not feel as comfortable or "in charge" as in the medical office. This may stem from the territorial anxiety of entering another's domain. By partially relinquishing the need to be in command of the situation, the physician may learn more about the family and thereby can render a more accurate diagnosis and plan more appropriate management. For example, the personal boundary issue in the family of one anorexic woman became vividly clear when the family physician and the author made a visit to the home of the mother during the patient's hospitalization. While she protested the fact that she could not control her daughter, she dutifully kept the daughter's cat, which literally destroyed her expensive furniture with its claws. Here we experienced firsthand the ambivalence that kept the family (and disease) going (26).

Metaphoric Considerations in Clinical Communication

From X-rays and ECGs to persons and families, all medicine hinges on interpretation (27). Interpretive processes and actions include: the selection of what to observe; the ruling in and ruling out of items in a differential diagnosis (from biomedical to psychiatric to familial); the explanation of the nature and prognosis of the problem to the patient (whether pathophysiological, etiological, interactional, or some other type); the decision about whether and how to intervene; and the later assessment of outcome. Explanations of what is wrong and how it came to be so, expectations of the type and style of treatment, and therapeutic goals are formulated not only by the physician but by all those involved in the clinical process, including family members. Kleinman refers to these influences as "explanatory models" (5).

Since people always use language to communicate with one another, the language tends to be confused with the nature of the reality we attempt to explain (28,29). Our organizing metaphors shape our perception of reality. For example, the metaphors of warfare, business, sports, and technology dominate medical thinking and influence clinical decision making and action. Military metaphors include "war on disease," "therapeutic armamentarium," "attack the illness," "therapeutic contract," and so on. These cultural metaphors are embodied in the classical medical model developed by "the microbe hunters" Pasteur, Koch, and Fleming (29–31). The astute clinician not only assesses and acts in terms of his/her framework, but also elicits and acknowledges the patient's and family's view of the illness, as well as their interpretation of cause, their expectations and beliefs about the problem, and their usual health-related behavior (self-medication, family-based decision making, lay referral process, use of alternative health care systems, etc.). Our usually implicit metaphors organize our thought and action (32,33). The physician who becomes more self-consciously aware of his/her own clinical orientation, and who actively elicits that of the patient and family, can frequently negotiate a common ground on which to proceed.

La Barre (34) wrote that "The family is the very root of all specifically human behaviors and institutions" (p. 164). This is as true for medicine as it is for law, morality, and religion. Physicians are often expected (and expect themselves) to play a psychological role that can be traced directly to the shaman–divine of Paleolithic times (35): the role of childhood's all-powerful parent. Moreover, as Benjamin (36) wrote, "Medicine, as anthropologists and theologians know, was born in magic and religion, and the doctor–priest–magician–parent unity that persists in the patient's unconscious cannot be broken" (p. 596). Only when the presence of magical wishes is acknowledged and addressed can its acting out in counterproductive ways be diminished.

The relationship between doctor and patient always risks being subverted by the patient's wish to receive, and the physician's desire to produce, a magical outcome (37). What separates scientific prescription from magical ritual is not just the pharmacologic content but also the meaning of *the act* to the participants in the clinical encounter. When an antibiotic or advice is presented or received as a "magic bullet," doctor or patient or both have forsaken the realm of science for magic. When scientific technique is manipulated for magical ends, what begins as overestimation of the physician's powers and goodness can plummet into disappointment, disillusionment, rage, paranoid accusation—and litigation. Patient compliance and satisfaction achieved by magical processes tend to be fleeting, ephemerally effective bursts of infantile wish fulfillment and imagined parental omnipotence (37). The healer who learns to forgo magic helps the patient to become healed or reconciled to life's irrevocable losses by first declining to comply with the patient's request for magic.

Much ineffective clinical communication derives from assumptions made about the meaning of what another person says. Physicians and patients often assume that the meanings of lay and medical terms are shared, when in fact they are often not. The full significance of a patient's words can be better appreciated if the physician avoids translating a patient's language into physician's meanings too quickly (38). When a patient describes a headache as "raging," for example, the patient's words are not only a guide to the severity of the pain, but also a potential cue to what the pain is about (rage). The clinician might inquire further about sources of frustration or anger, if not acutely during the headache, then when the pain has been attended to and relieved.

Even where the doctor, patient, and family appear to share the same religious, ethnic, or national culture, subtle differences in meaning and expectations may arise because of difference in age, sex, social class, and experience. For example, many midwestern physicians with whom I have worked are from wheat-farming families, so they are familiar with the values, priorities, and seasonal rounds of activities of their patients. Yet, as a result of their professionalization through years of medical school and residency, they quickly forget that during the harvest season (June to early July locally) virtually no one from farming families, save for small children, is brought in for medical care. The success of the harvest, fruition of a year's work, holds higher priority than health and life itself. As I reintroduce this family and cultural system to resident physicians, their anger toward and exasperation with these "noncompliant" patients frequently turns into an uncanny self-recognition and in turn not only greater compassion toward patients who share their same background yet who are now different, but also an effort to find ways of working within their system (16,39).

Patients and families often "hear" something far different from what the physician intends to communicate (and conversely). Patients and physicians often speak a different language even when they employ the same words. Americans equate "hypertension" with nervousness. Others who know it is high blood pressure believe it to be caused largely by "chronic external stress" (40). This belief may have considerable basis in fact, despite its being disdained by many physicians. The biomedical meanings of high blood pressure and low blood pressure differ markedly from the notions of "high blood" and "low blood" among many black patients (41). From the author's experience in the Bible Belt, many patients construe medical-sounding terms to have religious overtones. Thus, spinal meningitis becomes "Smilin' mighty Jesus," and fibroids on the uterus is heard as "fireballs on my Eucharist." Good preventive medicine includes asking the patient and family what they mean by a word or phrase, taking time to explain oneself in terms understandable to the patient and family, and checking to be sure they do in fact understand by asking them to explain it back to the physician. The primary care physician will often have to look for underlying wishes the patient may bring to the medical encounter, as well as the manifest complaint, if diagnosis is to be accurate and management therapeutic (37).

Time and Social Constraints upon Patient Care

Time is an often-overlooked dimension of the clinical relationship. The amount of time spent with a given patient (or family) is always a matter of choice, although that choice often *feels* as though it is out of the doctor's hands and carries certain costs. Several ingredients of a time-quota approach to patient care are: a certain standard of living to which the doctor and his/her family aspire; unconscious factors that influence the amount of time spent with a patient; in private practice, the substantial overhead that must be met; in corporate medicine, the tension between provider dedication to patient care and institutional pressure to keep the patient flow going; and frequent reminders from one's clinic staff that the waiting room is teeming while one is dawdling with a patient.

In many respects, physicians are trained to be overly responsible, to have difficulty saying "no" to patients or setting limits without feeling uncomfortable or inadequate. Setting time limits with patients can be a mature way of working with them, or it can be a thinly disguised maneuver to be free of the patient without having to say so. Alvah Cass, M.D., suggests saying to complicated patients, "You have an hour's worth of problems and I only have 15 minutes of time. What would you like to work on?" To avoid struggling to close the visit at the anticipated time, the physician can spell out the rules at the outset and anticipate the termination of the encounter without its being a source of contention.

Medical education and practice are expected to simultaneously (a) attend to the whole person and the wider psychosocial context, placing the patient's needs and sound clinical judgment above financial and institutional considerations, and (b) act in strict accordance with DRG, PSRO, PRO, and other guidelines while placing corporate and financial interests on a par with patient care. Traditions within the doctor–patient relationship are being challenged and reframed by many physicians' divided loyalties to patient care and to the institutions that support them through salaried positions, incentive bonuses for saving medical costs, etc.

As one family physician in his 60s complained: "We're getting into the era of DRGs. The issue is not quality of care. Just get them in and get them out—surgery, dead or alive. As fast as possible." A contradiction often arises between the institutional request for personal patient care ("patient first") and a structured set of impersonal behavioral constraints ("rules first"). The doctor who wants to aggressively cure disease, exercise independent clinical judgment, and be in charge of decision making and the direction of his/her medical career will likely feel constrained at times, not only by the patient and patient's family, but by the institutional and cultural restrictions of modern medicine.

The diagnosis is one component of the clinical relationship that extends beyond the family boundary into society. In many respects, American culture does not support the scientific and clinical interests of the doctor and the patient. Families, employers, and insurance companies are sometimes less genuinely interested in the welfare of the patient than is the doctor. For these, such diagnostic terms as "borderline personality," "hypertension," "sickle cell anemia," "cancer," "schizophrenia," "depression," and "AIDS" carry heavy stigmata and pass a moralistic social sentence on the patient (7,42–46). It may sometimes be as important for the physician to record a strategic diagnosis that has the *least* chance of hurting the patient socially as it is to formulate a scientific diagnosis of the patient's condition. To make strategic diagnoses, the physician needs to become intimately familiar with the patient's social environment. The clinical relationship, including the assessment process, is embedded in the larger social world, which reacts to diagnostic labels. If the patient is not to be unwittingly and unnecessarily condemned by the process of diagnosis, these repercussions need to be recognized.

The Use of One's Self in the Clinical Relationship

The physician's own self is a powerful tool of clinical assessment and treatment. By taking one's own emotional "temperature" in response to the patient—that is, how one feels while seeing the patient—one can gain a fairly accurate reading of the patient's or family's emotional "fever." One always understands another person better by being aware of one's own emotional response to that person. The clinical relationship is part of the healing process and can itself be variably therapeutic or antitherapeutic. It is antitherapeutic when the doctor attempts to defend him/herself against the painful material that the patient evokes. It is therapeutic when the doctor permits him/herself to empathize with another's illness, and thus to become better able to understand and respond to it (6–8). If the physician stays firmly planted in reality while eliciting and acknowledging the patient's wishes, he/she can help the patient work toward a more realistic understanding of diagnosis, management, and the future. The physician need not challenge a patient's (or a family's) unrealistic expectations or assumptions head on. Rather, as Gutheil, Bursztajn, and Brodsky (14) urge, it works better:

to empathize with the patient's wish for certainty and with its specific manifestations as understandable reactions to a difficult and painful situation. Explicit identification with the patient's fantasies is conveyed through such remarks as, "I wish I could give you a medication that was sure to have only positive effects" and "There is just no guarantee you'll live through this—I wish there were," which invite the patient to exchange idealization for identification. The patient can now approach the physician not as a childhood fantasy ideal but as another vulnerable human being facing—and hence, sharing—the same uncertainty. (p.50)

For example, difficulties arise in the treatment of patients with Adult Respiratory Distress Syndrome (ARDS), a disease with usually rapid, dramatic onset, and that frequently leads to death within days. To be therapeutic with these patients and their families, it is helpful for the physician to share with patient and family his/her own sense of shock and anger with the unexpected turn of events. The psychologic impact of unprepared-for worsening of the disease and the loss of the family member can be virtually the same for patient, family, physician(s), and staff alike. The whole system feels out of control. With patients/families with ARDS, as in other diseases, anger toward the physician and the medical system can be reduced if it is met with empathy instead of self-defense. The empathetic physician can acknowledge, accept, and help the patient and family deal with those powerful emotions of helplessness and rage that the physician may also feel.

Medical students are rarely taught how to use their intimate experiences with pain and death to listen to patients and to treat them better. Instead they usually learn how to avoid all forms of intimacy with patients. In the past decade some teachers of behavioral science to medical students and residents have encouraged dispassionate observation of selected verbal and nonverbal cues to infer what patients are thinking and feeling. American culture prizes efficiency, thus engendering the belief that one should be able to rapidly perform valid mental status examinations and psychiatric (family, social) histories. The complexity of deeply held values and beliefs and the difficulty patients have articulating them makes such "presto" results unlikely to be fully accurate. It is often assumed that accurate statements about a patient's inner state can be based solely upon direct observation (2). However, as Devereux (2) writes of the psychoanalyst: "In interpreting their reverberations within himself, the analyst professes to interpret *also* the unconscious of the patient" (p.304).

The same holds true for any physician who hopes to understand and to help the patient. Through the doctor's inspection of his/her own response to the patient or to a family interaction, the doctor is able to better understand the patient and thereby more accurately assess the facts, obtain more information, and design an effective intervention (2). One of the most powerful clinical instruments of assessment and intervention is the physician him/herself (2,7). The clinician's emotional response is a clue to what is going on with the patient and therefore a guide to an appropriate therapeutic response.

Clinical Example #5

A depressed, obese, hypertensive woman in her mid-20s visited the family medicine clinic for help with her hypertension and for counseling about her marriage. During one session, she said she resented her husband's ridiculing for being fat. "I can't think of losing weight until I feel better about myself," she protested. Her statement prompted an emotional response of sadness in the consultant, and the thought that there was something missing from her remark. The consultant used his feeling in response to her, saying: "There must be a lot that you don't like about yourself." She burst into tears. From this point she began to progress, exploring her own feelings and the reciprocal contributions of herself and her husband to their problems.

Content and Process in the Clinical Relationship

Most of medical education focuses on specific biomedical content, particularly on anatomy, physiology, biochemistry, and pathology. Renaissance philosopher Francis Bacon advocated the principle of *dissectio naturae,* the splitting of nature into its constituent, individual parts. Consonant with this empirical tradition of western science, medical education has long introduced medical students to a cadaver as their first patient, to be dissected into its inert structural components. In medical education, one deconstructs a person into an intricately related assortment of smaller and smaller elements and clearly delineated organ systems. It becomes very difficult to later put these Humpty Dumpty fragments back together into the person and life of which they are a part.

The biomedical model, instead of helping us to understand what is going on with an illness, may inadvertently dominate the thinking of both doctor and patient, i.e., the forest may not be seen for the trees. Medical students, presented a simplified world so that they can categorize phenomena and design interventions, may come to prefer the impersonal (cells, tissues, organs) to the personal (human). Patients can become secondary and their idiosyncracies may be seen as hindrances to the conquest of disease. The medical student is rewarded for displaying reductionistic acumen, which continues to be highly valued in traditional medical practice. From this limited perspective the patient becomes the battleground upon which the doctor's war is waged with disease; compliance becomes a battle of wills, one in which the patient is often seen as failing to uphold his/her part in the physician's fight to vanquish illness.

From a narrow viewpoint, the main issues are whether and how to perform a certain procedure or prescribe a medication. Physicians generally think that patients share their biomedical style of reasoning and problem solving; to a variable degree they do, but perhaps not to the degree physicians assume. Physicians usually make little effort to elicit the patient's expectations, values, and constraints, which strongly influence subsequent compliance with medical advice (5). Doctors are also trained to mistrust and discount their own feelings and intuitions, rather than using them as clinical instruments in patient care. This is unfortunate, since the *process* of the relationships between doctor and patient, family, and clinical-administrative staff heavily influences clinical outcomes, including patient satisfaction (1,5,7,8,15,47).

Clinical Example #6

At a recent Family Medicine case conference, the resident summarized a 78-year-old patient's recent medical history of transient ischemic attacks, acute small bowel obstruction, and acute cerebrovascular accidents. These problems had forced the patient, who had been living alone in good health, to enter a nursing home. After briefly presenting a biomedical problem list, the resident spent about 25 minutes discussing technical issues in carotid angiography (medical indications, anatomy, test procedure, and interpretation). The author commented: "You have just summarized from a biomedical viewpoint what *could* be done. I wonder whether you might address the issues of cost considerations versus considerations of patient care. Furthermore, how do the patient and the family feel about these various tests?" The resident responded elusively that there is "uncertainty whether she is having TIA. . . . you need to make the diagnosis to clarify what's going on with the patient, even if you're not able to do surgery." The resident and faculty group did not press for more consideration of psychosocial issues.

The author mentioned the work of Erik Erikson, who in the 1940s conceptualized a developmental scheme that included issues of "integrity" versus "despair" (48) in this final phase of the life cycle. Dealing with these issues involves the aging person asking him/herself, "Has it all been worthwhile? What have I lived for?" The author urged that the patient and her family be given a chance to talk about their feelings, and suggested that the physician help the family adjust to the patient's changes and begin to say good-bye to her. The conference concluded shortly thereafter.

While the technical discussion was interesting and pertinent, the author felt that dwelling on it to the exclusion of psychosocial issues allowed the resident, if not also the group, to avoid dealing with the upsetting emotional issues of limits on the physician's ability to intervene and control disease, and the patient and family's coping with disability and impending death.

The doctor's availability and compassion for one or more family members leads to growing feelings of mutual trust that often solidify as a physician intervenes successfully in the patient's and family's life. These elements of time and relationship are not reducible to specific biomedical content. Consider the anorexic teenager discussed earlier in Clinical Example #2. Only by working with several combinations of family members over several months were we able to make good diagnostic and therapeutic sense out of the multiple problems in various family members—anorexia nervosa, gastrointestinal pain, headache, and depression. This family, we learned, was terrified of the prospect of separation and loss, and expressed this core issue through an assortment of symptoms. Continuing comprehensive care that included an empathetic clinical relationship facilitated discovery of this deeper issue. It also helped the family confront and begin to work on the destructive underlying dynamic.

The ability to persevere with a patient, to note and reflect upon a patient's anger rather than retreat or retaliate to preserve self-esteem, and to understand the patient's environment—these are skills that are every bit as important as knowing all the clinically relevant facts about digoxin. Attention to the ebb and flow of the clinical relationship over time is as important as attention to the biomedical details of diagnosis and intervention (49). The physician who takes an interest in the patient's life situation will obtain cues about the patient's readiness for change and will thus be able to work within the patient's context. In primary care medical practice, continuity and comprehensiveness of care are two of the keys for taking good care of patients. For many doctors, a personal relationship with patient and family over time is more rewarding than the successful mastery of technical procedures. Procedures tend to become dull with increasing familiarity, while people are ever fascinating to the caring physician.

Conclusion

In this chapter the systemic nature of the clinical relationship has been explored. For purposes of discussion, components of the clinical system were artificially grouped into persons (who?), institutions, occasions, and places (where?), and issues (what?). The clinical relationship with patient and family is embedded in a wide variety of meanings, relationships, and contexts. In each new patient interaction, recognizing the major factors that affect the clinical relationship promotes a truly scientific and therapeutic process. Neglecting to attend to the clinical relationship leads to a mechanistic and merely pragmatic approach that works only to some degree in the short run with some problems. The highly competent physician becomes a curious and competent observer of self and the individual who is ill, as well as of the biomedical disease. The clinician who understands the "who, what, and where" of the illness is able to diagnose more accurately and plan more effective management.

Acknowledgment. The author gratefully acknowledges the diligent editing and typing on this manuscript by Margaret A. Stein, M.A.

References

1. Balint M: The Doctor, His Patient and the Illness. New York, International Universities Press, 1957.
2. Devereux G: From Anxiety to Method in the Behavioral Sciences. The Hague, Mouton, 1967.
3. Szasz TS, Hollender MH: A contribution to the philosophy of medicine: The basic models of the doctor–patient relationship, in Millon T (ed): Medical Behavioral Science. Philadelphia, Saunders, 1975.
4. Froelich RE, Bishop FM: Clinical Interviewing Skills, ed 3. St. Louis, Mosby, 1977.
5. Kleinman A: Patients and Healers in the Context of Culture: An Exploration of the Borderland Between Anthropology, Medicine, and Psychiatry. Los Angeles, CA, University of California Press, 1980.

6. Katz J: The Silent World of Doctor and Patient. New York, Free Press, 1984.
7. Stein HF: The Psychodynamics of Medical Practice: Unconscious Factors in Patient Care. Berkeley, University of California Press, 1985.
8. Stein HF, Apprey M: Context and Dynamics in Clinical Knowledge. Monograph Series in Ethnicity, Medicine, and Psychoanalysis, vol 1. Charlottesville, VA, University Press of Virginia, 1985.
9. Doherty WJ, Baird MA: Family Therapy and Family Medicine: Toward the Primary Care of Families. New York, The Guilford Press, 1983.
10. Bronowski J: Science and Human Values. New York, Harper and Row, 1956.
11. Thomas L: Late Night Thoughts on Listening to Mahler's Ninth Symphony. New York, The Viking Press, 1983.
12. Whitehead AN: Science and the Modern World. New York, Macmillan, 1925.
13. Richtsmeier AJ, Waters DB: Somatic symptoms as family myth. Am J Dis Child 1984;138:855–857.
14. Gutheil TJ, Bursztajn H, Brodsky A: Malpractice prevention through the sharing of uncertainty. N Engl J Med 1984;311:49–51.
15. Schwartzman HB, Kneifel AW, Barbera-Stein L, Gaviria E: Children, families, and mental health service organizations: Cultures in conflict. Hum Org 1984;43:297–306.
16. Stein HF: The annual cycle and the cultural nexus of health care behavior among Oklahoma wheat farming families. Culture, Med Psychiatry 1982;6:81–99.
17. Stein HF, Fox D: Work as family: Occupational relationships and social transference, In Stein HF, Apprey M: Context and Dynamics in Clinical Knowledge. Monograph Series in Ethnicity, Medicine, and Psychoanalysis, vol 1. Charlottesville, VA, University Press of Virginia, 1985.
18. Stein HF: The case study method as a means of teaching significant context in family medicine. Fam Med 1983;15:163–167.
19. Stein HF: The boundary of the symptom: *Whose* death and dying? Fam Syst Med 1984;2(2):188–194.
20. Earley LW, von Mering O: Growing old the outpatient way. Am J Psychiatry 1969;125:963–967.
21. Wilmer HA: Transference to a medical center: A cultural dimension in healing. Calif Med 1962;96:173–180.
22. Crouch MA: Working with one's own family: Another path for professional development. Fam Med (in press).
23. deMause L: Foundations of Psychohistory. New York, Creative Roots, 1982.
24. Schmidt DD: When is it helpful to convene the family? J Fam Pract 1983;16:967–973.
25. Galazka SS, Eckert JK: Diabetes mellitus from the inside out: Ecological perspectives on a chronic disease. Fam Syst Med 1984;2(1):28–36.
26. Stein HF, Wilson TA: "How could I eat uncaring food?": From identified patient to family pathology, In Stein HF: The Psychodynamics of Medical Practice: Unconscious Factors in Patient Care. Berkeley, University of California Press, 1985.
27. Good BJ, Good M-JD: The meaning of symptoms: A cultural hermeneutic model for clinical practice, in Eisenberg L, Kleinman A (eds): The Relevance of Social Science for Medicine. Dordrecht, Holland, D. Reidel, 1981, pp 165–196.

28. Stein HF, Apprey M: From Metaphor to Meaning: Papers in Psychoanalytic Anthropology. Monograph Series in Ethnicity, Medicine, and Psychoanalysis, vol 2. Charlottesville, VA, University Press of Virginia, 1985.
29. Stein HF, Hill RF: American medicine and the enchanted machine (guest ed). Contin Educ Fam Physician 1984;19:428–430.
30. Burnside JW: Medicine and war—A metaphor. JAMA 1983;249:2091.
31. Caster JH, Gatens-Robinson E: Metaphor in medicine (letter to the editor). JAMA 1983;250:1841.
32. Ransom DC: Resistance: Family- or therapist-generated, in Gurman AS (ed): Questions and Answers in the Practice of Family Therapy, vol 2. New York, Brunner/Mazel, 1982, pp 3–10.
33. Wilden A: System and Structure: Essays in Communication and Exchange, ed 2. London, Tavistock, 1980.
34. La Barre W: Family and symbol, in Wilbur G, Muensterberger W (eds): Psychoanalysis and Culture: Essays in Honor of Geza Roheim. New York, International Universities Press, 1951, pp 156–167.
35. La Barre W: Shamanic origins of religion and medicine. J Psychedelic Drugs 1979;11(1–2):7–11.
36. Benjamin WW: Healing by the fundamentals. N Engl J Med 1984;111:595–597.
37. Boyer LB: Approaching cross-cultural psychotherapy. J Psychoanal Anthropol 1983;6:237–245.
38. Friedman WH, Jelly E, Jelly P: Language of the patient with a raging headache. J Fam Pract 1979;8:401–402.
39. Stein HF, Pontious JM: Family and beyond: The larger context of noncompliance. Fam Syst Med1985;3(2):179–189.
40. Blumhagen D: Hyper-Tension: A folk illness with a medical name. Culture, Med Psychiatry 1980;4:197–227.
41. Snow LF: Traditional health beliefs and practices among lower class black Americans. West J Med 1983;139:820–828.
42. Goffman E: Stigma: Notes on the Management of Spoiled Identity. Englewood Cliffs, NJ, Prentice-Hall, 1963.
43. Phillips JR: Mental health and SCA: A psycho-social approach. Urban Health 1973;2(6):36–40.
44. Sontag S: Illness as Metaphor. New York, Vintage (Random House), 1979.
45. Stein HF: Rehabilitation and chronic illness in American culture: The cultural psychodynamics of a medical and social problem. J Psychol Anthropol 1979;2:153–176.
46. Stein HF: Illness as Metaphor, by Susan Sontag (review) J Psychol Anthropol 1980;3:33–38.
47. Korsch BM, Negrette VF: Doctor–patient communication. Sci Am 1972;227:66–74.
48. Erikson EH: Childhood and Society, ed 2. New York, Norton, 1963.
49. Stein HF: The ebb and flow of the clinical relationship, In Stein HF, Apprey M: Context and Dynamics in Clinical Knowledge. Monograph Series in Ethnicity, Medicine, and Psychoanalysis, vol 1. Charlottesville, VA, University Press of Virginia, 1985.

CHAPTER 3

Family Systems Theory In Medical Practice

Leonard Roberts

In medical practice some patient presentations are not adequately explained by the usual textbook descriptions of pathophysiology. Understanding the interactions in the patient's family, for example, is essential for evaluating and managing the presenting problem in a family where a 10-year-old with asthma seems to be the focus of a power struggle between parents; or when the parents in a reconstituted (step) family appear overly involved with an 11-year-old with headaches; or when a 30-year-old woman with increasingly frequent headaches feels isolated from her working husband, overwhelmed by the demands of caring for three small children, and fails to recognize the impact of her mother's death upon her life.

Problems such as parent–child conflicts, alcohol abuse, sexual dysfunction, and psychosomatic illness often present with one family member as the identified patient, but the whole family is involved in the illness (1–4). Exactly how the family is involved and what constitutes proper management may not be clear. It is helpful (as explained later) for the clinician to formulate a diagnosis that locates the problem in the context of the family and the circumstances under which the symptoms occur.

The relationships between family dynamics and the health and illness of family members are studied in the disciplines of sociology, medicine, family therapy, social work, psychology, and anthropology. Family therapists and other systems-oriented clinicians have written a great deal about the family and illness (5–13). How the principles of family systems theories can best be applied in medical practice is the subject of this chapter (4,14–20). The first example emphasizes the added dimension of understanding that such an approach affords the physician.

Clinical Example #1

Mrs. Jones, presented Nicholas, her 11-year-old son, for a checkup. Mrs. Jones told the physician that Nick had severe asthma, which required numerous emergency room visits and changes in medications. They have changed doctors several times because of his "delicate condition," according to Mrs. Jones. She requested that Nick be placed on "steroids" immediately. She stated that he has always been her "sick child" and that the three older boys were never this much of a problem. While Mrs. Jones described Nick as a sick patient, he smiled and bowed his head.

After Mrs. Jones left the room, the clinician talked with Nick and discovered a pattern of symptoms. Nick noted that his worst symptoms often occurred when his father was angry and/or vocally critical of him. He also thought his asthma worsened when his father and mother began to argue. While discussing these issues with the clinician, Nick appeared somewhat sad and afraid, and his breathing was more rapid and shallow.

Later that day, the clinician received a telephone call from Mr. Jones, who said he just learned of the office visit by Mrs. Jones and Nick and wanted to set the record straight. He stated that there was nothing seriously wrong with Nick, except for laziness, and that his mother was overprotective. He said that he has told Nicholas over and over to just calm down. Mr. Jones also described Nicholas as bullheaded and uncooperative.

Later in the day, a second telephone call came from a friend of the Jones family who expressed concern about Mr. Jones' drinking pattern. The family friend said Mr. Jones denied being an alcoholic, but that during the past two years he had become quite verbally abusive at home during frequent drinking binges. The friend was concerned that Mr. and Mrs. Jones were discussing sending Nick to military school so that he could learn better self-discipline.

The Jones family example challenges the description of Nick as the only patient and asthma as the only problem. What diagnoses encompass the medical problem and its context? Is it accurate to describe Nick's problem as just asthma, and does such a diagnosis acknowledge the situation surrounding his symptoms? What will it take for Nick's asthma symptoms to improve? Should a plan of management include not only an optimal regimen of medications, but also attention to the family interaction pattern, which seems to influence the symptoms? If Nick felt less anxiety and were not caught in the middle of a parental struggle, would his symptoms improve and the need for medications decrease? How is Mr. Jones' drinking behavior related to the whole issue and how can it be addressed effectively? How is Mrs. Jones maintaining the cycle of symptoms and office visits? There are many reasons why family systems theories should be of interest to physicians. The above example touched on a few of these; other reasons are explained below.

Rationale for Learning How to Work with Families

Families Are the Settings in Which Most Patients Live

Most individuals are products of family interactions—genetic and social. Families are complex organizations with observable behavior patterns and structure (such as when and how to eat, sleep, play, work, express emotion, etc.). Most patients are active members of family systems, with on-going interactions with other members of their nuclear and/or extended families. In caring for patients, most physicians must deal with the family to some extent. To effectively relate to and work with other family members, it is helpful for the clinician to understand how families work and how they get into trouble (17,18,20).

Families Affect Health and Illness

Although the importance of the relationship between a presenting patient and the patient's family has been long recognized (1,2,4,9), it has recently been more widely researched and discussed (3,14–26). Table 3.1 summarizes articles that explore the relationships between family dynamics and individual illness.

The family may contribute to the production and/or maintenance of symptoms as much as or more than any other factor—e.g., the asthma attacks in Clinical Example #1, or tension headaches in one member of the nice couple who never have a cross word. To reach a more complete diagnosis and understanding (as opposed to just a diagnostic label) the physician needs to explore the symptoms in terms of the family system. To diagnose Nick, for instance, as just an adolescent having asthma is inadequate because it ignores other important factors. Besides physiologic predisposition to bronchospasm, medication responses, and activity level, individual psychologic factors and family dynamics influence Nick's course (20,27–29). Management based on an incomplete understanding is less likely to be effective than a plan that addresses all the important factors (12,29).

Although there has been a great deal of research in the field, there is no one coherent family systems theory. Instead, several theories have evolved, each emphasizing different aspects of family interaction. Table 3.2 lists several theories that have been studied and applied in a medical context. Each of these theories highlights a particular aspect of family dynamics that may be useful, depending upon the presenting problem. Parent–child relationship issues that seem to exacerbate asthma, for example, may be best conceptualized and managed by employing the structural family theory. Marital discord complicated by alcohol or substance

TABLE 3.1. Articles addressing family dynamics and illness.

Study	Results
Minuchin et al. (11, 12, 29–31)	Studied families with adolescents who had diabetes, asthma, or anorexia nervosa.
	Described characteristics of family organization that produced or maintained symptoms; designed management that addressed family aspects of illness.
Steinglass (37)	Studied families with at least one alcoholic member and proposed working models for clinicians dealing with such families.
Pfeffer (53)	Studied the family systems of hospitalized suicidal children and described characteristics of such systems.

TABLE 3.1. *Continued*

Study	Results
Widmer et al. (49)	Studied depressed patients in a family practice setting. Noted pain, psychosomatic and anxiety complaints in a significant proportion of relatives of depressed patients.
Cleveland (22)	Studied families with a drug-dependent member. Analyzed roles of siblings and suggested clinical intervention.
Ackerman et al. (21)	Reviewed data on 34 adolescent and preadolescent patients with peptic ulcer disease and noted 10 had encountered separation or loss within 12 months of the onset of illness (matched to 24 appendectomy patients as controls). Results suggest that a recent separation or loss may be associated with the onset of peptic ulcer disease in predisposed persons.
Meyer and Haggerty (35)	Studied families and noted increased incidence of streptococcal infection within 2 weeks of family crises.
Huygen (4)	Studied and recorded office consultations of family members in over 30 years of family practice. Noted family patterns of illness, response, involvement, and impact of illness upon the family over time.
Schmidt (55)	Presents case example and review of literature concerning the occurrence of illness after the death of a family member and explores issue of impaired immunity following such a stressful life event.
Marshall and Neill (34)	Examined the effects in the marriage of 12 patients who underwent intestinal bypass surgery for extreme obesity. Noted marked disruption in marriage relationship with conflict in the areas of sexuality and dependence/independence issues theorized to be the result of changes postsurgery (loss of morbid obesity).
Hadley et al. (7)	Studied 90 families in an outpatient facility and noted onset of clinically significant symptoms with the addition or loss of a family member. The changes and distress generated by loss or addition of a family member are theorized to be related to the onset of such symptoms.
Stanton (52)	Studied families with a member abusing drugs and conceptualized behaviors in terms of family patterns.
Parkes (48)	Studied medical records of widows and found increased incidence of morbidity and mortality after the loss of spouse.
Medalie et al. (56)	Studied multiple risk factors for ischemic heart disease in 10,000 men. Found perceived degree of support of family (marital) relationship to be directly related to morbidity and mortality.

TABLE 3.2. Comparison of family systems theories.

Theory	Author	Emphasis	Approach question
Structural	Minuchin	Understanding individual behavior requires understanding the structure of the family.	Who has power over what (or whom) in this family? Identify subsystems, boundaries, and rules.
Strategic	Haley, Erickson	Problem behavior is an integral part of family interactional patterns and serves a function.	What is the problem behavior? What function does it serve? What pattern supports it? What will it take to change?
Multigenerational	Bowen	Individual behavior depends upon family myths, traditions, and emotional interconnectedness among generations.	How might the family system be preventing individuation? What family beliefs/explanations may influence this patient in this setting? How is this person connected to the family?
Communication	Satir, Jackson	Individual behavior is understood in terms of communication patterns.	Who is saying what to whom? What might be said differently or more clearly? What conflicts are accentuated or symbolized by the presenting problem?
Reciprocity	Lidz, Jackson	Interpersonal exchange builds the trust that is essential for family relationship stability. Behavior is understood in terms of *quid pro quo* balance. Present behavior is supported by the system and change will unbalance the system.	Who wants what from whom? How may they get it in a less problem-producing way? What can they exchange for it?

abuse might fit best with the exchange or communication theories. Though no single theory may work best for all cases, all of the theories have useful concepts to help the physician understand the family.

Finally, all families have a heritage that influences the illness and the family's response to illnesses. The family with a presenting symptomatic member is a mixture of family rituals, beliefs, and roles influenced by previous generations of the family (5,19). People *learn* within this family context how to interpret and respond to symptoms, i.e., when to call the doctor, what medicines to take before consultation, how to act when sick, and how and when to ask for help (7,10,11,14). At times families may complicate illness by overinvolvement (creating a cardiac cripple, for example). At other times families impair the health of their members by underinvolvement (child neglect). To manage patient problems effectively, the physician must learn to discern not only what the symptoms mean to the patient, but also how the family may be helping produce or maintain symptoms by their pattern of response. In Clinical Example #1, Nick's symptoms signaled his reaction to the distressing family interaction patterns, and the family's response (unified concern about him) probably reinforced Nick's tendency to have an asthma attack when his anxiety level increased. Such a response pattern may be strongly influenced by the experiences and beliefs about asthma that Nick's parents hold from their own families of origin. It would not be unusual to find other members in their family background that either had some type of lung trouble (like Nick) and/or were alcoholic (like Mr. Jones) (4,9).

Illness in this context depends not only upon the tissue pathology, but also on the learned responses of both the individual and the family to such pathology. Such learned responses are influenced by the beliefs and experiences of previous generations, regardless of how appropriate such responses are to the current situation. Two patients with the same diagnostic label but in different families (or even the sam family) require different management, not only because of individual differences, but also because of differences in family patterns of response to illness (being an asthmatic oldest child is different from being an asthmatic youngest child, even in the same family) (12,29).

Knowledge of Family Systems Aids Early Diagnosis

Physicians also benefit from learning about family systems because they learn to spot opportunities to prevent illness and dysfunction through early diagnosis and intervention (12,16,30). The physician can learn to routinely assess patients' family systems and anticipate which (and when) families are at increased risk for illness or emotional upset and act accordingly. The routine physical examination, for example, is a good time to inquire about predictable issues of the family life cycle, as well as a time to inquire about habits and meal times. The well baby visit is an opportunity to assess the family's response to the birth of a child (overinvolvement, underinvolvement, effect on couple bond, etc.). The hospital visit to a terminally ill patient is also a visit to a *family* with a terminally ill member.

Several frameworks are particularly adaptable to the medical encounters among doctor, patient, and family. Minuchin described the characteristics of family organization that produce and/or maintain psychosomatic symptoms and illness (11,12,31). Healthy and unhealthy family systems have been described, along with methods of assessment (32,33). Family life cycle transition periods (see Chapter 4) and stressful life events (divorce, death of a family member, job change, etc.) are accompanied by an increased incidence of illness (4,21,34,35) and an increase in the number of consultations with a physician (4,25). Once dysfunction, psychosomatogenic qualities, and predictable (and unpredictable) life stress events are recognized, the physician can learn how to respond accordingly (further evaluation, counseling, referral, scheduled visits, etc.). Later in the chapter a process of evaluating a family system is described to help the physician recognize families at increased risk.

Understanding Family Systems Helps Avoid Entanglement

Perhaps most importantly, learning about family dynamics can help the physician avoid frustrating and time-consuming entanglements with patients and their families. Such imbroglios can occur more easily if the physician is unaware of family systems effects upon the illness (19,20,31,36). In Clinical Example #1, for instance, one can imagine how frustrating the combination of continued symptoms, numerous emergency room visits, and multiple admissions could be for both a conscientious clinician and Nick's family. Add to this the clinician's feeling of impotence and frustration, and a vicious cycle continues that is inefficient, expensive, and time-consuming for everyone involved. It is easy to understand how even the strongest of clinician–patient relationships may become strained beyond its capacity to tolerate anxiety, frustration, and anger. An accurate assessment and understanding of the pattern of events would have prevented or at least interrupted the cycle of events.

Understanding more about families and illness also leads to a better physician awareness of why it is more difficult for him/her to work with some family members than others (2,19). Suppose, for instance, the physician in Clinical Example #1 found it extremely hard to deal with Nick's father or Nick himself. Such frustration might be expected if Nick's father evokes the ambivalence and/or helplessness the physician feels in dealing with his own alcoholic father, or if Nick reminds him of his own brother with asthma. Operating under such masked pressure, clinicians may unwittingly limit their own effectiveness in several ways: (a) by forming an alliance with one family member against another ("I told you the doctor would see it my way"); (b) by giving advice without understanding all the factors involved ("Just relax, Nick, and take your medicine."); (c) by spending too much time correcting the wrong factors ("juggling medicines'' in a person whose asthma is very sensitive to distress, without designing a plan to deal with the sources of distress); (d) by becoming overly involved in a struggle with one family member; or (e) by assuming too much responsibility for Nick's symptoms and becoming angry or sarcastic when Nick doesn't improve ("Nick is a crock. His father is a drunk. What do you expect?") (2,5,18). Drawing upon one's knowledge of the family dynamics and their relationship to symptoms allows the clinician to evaluate the whole picture in the context of the family and design a more appropriate strategy.

Characteristics of Family Systems

Wholeness

Wholeness means that the family, as an entity, has its own character, communication style, strengths, and weaknesses. Each individual family member, for instance, may function competently in his/her respective occupation—effectively employing skills for solving problems, communicating, and negotiating. These same people as a family unit, however, may not do well with problem solving, communicating, or negotiating, unable to use at home the same skills required at work. This becomes important clinically because of predisposing factors that affect risk of illness (11,21,25,35) and behavior patterns and emotional intensity that affect the course of illness (2,14,17,27). Understanding alcoholism, for example, as a family with an alcoholic member leads to a different conceptualization and approach than singling out the symptomatic member (20,37).

Wholeness, then, refers to the family as a group and its distinctive characteristics. What are its strengths and weaknesses? How adaptable is this family? How does it handle crisis or conflict? Although research demonstrates no perfect family system, it does identify advantages and disadvantages of particular types of family systems (9,11,31,38).

Homeostasis

Family homeostasis is the dynamic equilibrium of the family (9). Much that occurs with one family member affects other members in some way. If one member becomes ill, for instance, then the other members compensate, thus restoring a state of equilibrium. Depending on the seriousness and duration of the illness, the new equilibrium may involve little or great differences from the preillness balance.

Homeostatic factors may complicate health issues for individual members. For instance, changes in the family generated by a new eating plan, or by a person's feeling better as a result of weight loss, may be resisted by other members (34). The clinical relevance is significant because, otherwise, physicians attribute ineffectiveness (in the weight loss example) to ''lack of will power'' or other mistaken assumptions about the patient.

While the concept of homeostasis is useful to emphasize the interrelatedness of family members, it can be misleading and is not without controversy. One may infer incorrectly that homeostatic families are in a static equilibrium, i.e., that stability means inactivity. This is misleading because, in fact, family systems are constantly in motion. Families are responding to continual challenges from within (individual needs, illness, family life cycle events) and from without (societal expectations, economic pressures, and so on).

Another tempting but false assumption is that, when a family is in equilibrium, it is healthy—that homeostasis per se is the ideal. Again, this is misleading because a well-developed, stable system may be an unhealthy system (e.g., a child abuse family system or an alcoholic system). Healthy family systems tend to be broadly stable, and changing over time because of their ability to receive stimuli and adapt (6,32,39).

It follows, then, that not all upsets to family systems are undesirable. In fact, some are inevitable and essential for growth and development (maturation of children and adults, disruption of a drug abuse system, or intervention in a child abuse family system). Therapy can be viewed as either an aid to returning to a more desirable equilibrium or an intervention that disrupts an unhealthy but stable state. The basic question for the physician with respect to homeostasis is, "How is this symptom or illness stabilizing and/or disrupting the system?"

Family Dynamics

Family dynamics is a general term for patterns of actions and interactions among the members in a family system and the effect of such interactions on the family unit. The portion of an interaction that is observable is only part of the dynamic. The meaning of a certain interaction is sometimes imperceptible to the clinician, but the meaning may be the key to understanding the sequence of events (a loud laugh or headache may mean "I don't want to talk about alcohol."). The clinician who can observe and note the interactions of the family, getting a sense of how each member interprets interactions, is better able to understand and predict what symptoms are likely to appear under certain conditions. (What is the identified patient saying about or for the family with these symptoms?)

Family Roles and Rules

Each family operates with certain rules or norms of behavior. There are overt, consciously defined rules (curfew, meal time, household responsibilities), and thousands of unconscious ones (how and when to eat, sleep, play, work, communicate, express emotion, express sexuality, resolve differences; how to be a wife, husband, son, daughter, sister, brother) (1,40). Family roles and rules emerge as patterns of behavior of the current family but are derived from the beliefs, rituals, and emotional connectedness of previous generations. Each spouse brings his/her own heritage into the family. As the family adds members, a distinctive collage of behaviors evolves that expresses and reflects the interrelatedness with previous generations. Family myths and traditions often repeat generations so that the physician may recognize such tendencies early and respond accordingly (e.g., anxiety in the family of a 46-year-old man whose father died at 47 of a heart attack; tolerant family attitudes about obesity and weight control) (4,19,37,38,41).

Some family rules can be deduced from observable behaviors that form a predictable pattern for the observant clinician (1,40). In clinical practice, perceptive physicians have long observed such family patterns of behavior (1,4,7,14,35). Some families, for instance, wait until they are deathly ill to contact a physician; others call at the slightest problem. All families have observable patterns of behavior that can help the clinician understand and predict the sequence of events. (How will this family complicate patient A's recovery from his heart attack? How will they aid his recovery?)

Subsystems

Subsystems are the smaller units within the family, such as the parental subunit, the sibling subunit, the spouse subunit, or a parent–child subunit. A subsystem (or subunit) may be an individual or any combination of individual members that is less than the whole family system. Subsystems are identified by what they do (function) and who participates in them (membership). For instance, the parental subunit has an executive function (parenting) and typically is composed of the two adult spouses (or a single parent) (20,31). Awareness of subunits enables the clinician to dissect out how the family works, who is allied with whom, who is locked into struggle with whom, who is likely to be caught in the middle and who is likely to feel the most distress (11,31).

Boundaries

The rules that govern who participates in a subsystem (membership) and what that subsystem does (function) are the boundaries. The marital subunit, for instance, is typically composed of two adult spouses and ideally provides for their mutual growth and support. This can be clearly differentiated from the child subunit by both membership and function. Intrafamily boundaries are generally of two types—generational (parent–child) and individual (5,11,12,31).

If the boundaries of the subunits are not well defined, then the family is described as enmeshed. This family may describe itself as a "real close family," but it is, in fact, too close. The individuals are emotionally "stuck together" or fused. Little privacy, individuality, and differentness are allowed. Conflict may be avoided and repressed at times and raging out of control at other times, but is hardly ever resolved (5,11,12,31). Minuchin described such families and their propensity for producing symptomatic members because of the emotional intensity (11,12,31).

If, on the other hand, the subunits are sharply demarcated and the boundaries are overly rigid, then the family may be described as disengaged, i.e., isolated individual units instead of a family unit. These families hardly function as what most people consider families at all, but may more accurately be described as individuals sharing a roof. Whereas the problem in an enmeshed family is overinvolvement in each other's lives, the opposite extreme, underinvolvement, characterizes the disengaged family. There is little or no overt involvement between family members, and little or no mutual support and understanding (no one visits a sick family member in the hospital). The members of disengaged families may well have a lot of underground emotional intensity, however, that manifests as illness or dysfunction (5,11,12,40).

In between the two extremes is a wide range of functional family systems with well-defined but flexible boundaries. In these families it is relatively clear who comprises the parental subunit, the marital subunit, and the sibling subunit, and there is no cutoff or isolation of subunits from each other. This arrangement allows both individual identity and mutual involvement. One can interact appropriately across boundaries and function and grow effectively. Family members are able to adjust their emotional closeness and distance so that they can continue to meet their own and each other's needs despite changing circumstances (1,5,18,32,33).

Adaptability

The ability of a family to adapt to life events (temporary or permanent loss of a member, sickness, addition of a member, etc.) determines its survival as a family, and heavily influences its likelihood of becoming a dysfunctional or unhealthy family (11,12,17,20,30,38,42). Probably the most common example in primary care is the ability of the family to adapt to a spouse becoming ill. The other spouse may have to assume the missing role, such as a woman working outside the home after her husband's heart attack. The change in his role may be very hard for the husband/father to accept. In a family with poor adaptability, the father's reaction will influence his recovery and the family's function. If he is resentful, depressed, and demanding, another member (a child or the working mother) may present to the physician with headaches or depression as a result. In a more adaptable family in this situation, the father might ease the impact of change by doing some of the housework and/or enjoy learning to play the guitar or cook. The mother might gain great fulfillment from a midlife discovery of her latent talent in a satisfying job. The ability of each to realize and make individual changes depends upon other members' ability and willingness to adapt.

Communication

Families that communicate effectively appear to also function more effectively, and with less distress (1–3,20,31,42). Communication (verbal and nonverbal) is a major feedback mechanism for the family. It is how one member learns what the other members expect, want, like, and so forth. Dysfunctional or unhealthy family systems typically exhibit masked and indirect communication, while more effective family systems communicate clearly and directly (1,33,39).

Communication and triangulation in families have been studied and described by Bowen and others (5,11,43). Triangulation refers to interactions among three people or between two people about a third person or object. The pattern tends to occur when anxiety is heightened, and it functionally prevents resolution of conflict. Spouses, through overfocusing on a child, may, for example, avoid both intimacy and possible conflict. Triangulation by spouses often channels the conflicts and negative communication through a child, creating some real difficulties for both child and family. One spouse may be essentially saying, for instance, "I don't like the way you do things" to the other spouse by competing for the child's attention or support. Such a pattern can form a stable triangle, which places the child in a double bind. In order to please one parent, the child must choose against the other (Nick in Clinical Example #1). If the child is susceptible to such distress, symptoms will appear and recur as long as the unresolved conflict that maintains the distress continues to smolder (11,12).

People may also triangulate communication with the clinician or family through symptoms. A migraine headache may mean "Take care of me!", "Go away!", and/or "You make me sick!" It may direct attention from the underlying tension-producing conflict. The physician who can determine if there is a message in the symptoms, and if that message or conflict is connected with the symptoms, will find such cases less frustrating to manage. Less time will be spent discussing and treating the triangulated symptom and more time addressing the unresolved conflict (2,4,5,11,14,19,20).

Clinical Application of Family System Principles

Clinical Example #2

Mr. Britt is a 45-year-old businessman who presented with the chief complaint of chest pain described as "burning in the middle of my chest." The pain had been constantly present for several weeks, but not getting any worse from the first day. The pain did not radiate and was not exercise related, nor was it accompanied by sweating or weakness. Ingestion of food sometimes relieved the pain and occasionally exacerbated it. He had experienced nausea without vomiting. He had no history of melena, early AM burning, or early satiety, diarrhea, or change in bowel habit. Mr. Britt experienced a similar pain several years ago and was told he had only a hiatal hernia on an upper gastrointestinal series (UGI).

Past Medical History: His health has been generally very good. His only hospitalization was several years ago for the work-up of similar pain. Besides the UGI series mentioned above, he had a barium enema, electrocardiogram, and blood work that were all normal.

Review of Systems: No other symptoms.

Habits: He had smoked 1–2 packs of cigarettes for 20 years. He drank "to excess occasionally," becoming very intoxicated, several times a year. He described himself as a binge drinker.

Family History: Neither of his parents are living. He believed his father had high blood pressure and heart trouble, although he lived into his late 70s. His only sibling, a brother, died of myocardial infarction at age 54. His mother he knew little about, as she died while he was an infant. He had been married for 25 years and had two children, a 16-year-old daughter and a 22-year-old son, both of whom lived at home, although the son attended college (living on campus during the school year).

Physical Examination: Mr. Britt appeared to be in generally good health and his exam was unremarkable. His mental status exam revealed that he sounded moderately depressed and frustrated about his symptoms and exhibited a rather sad affect. He did smile occasionally, however.

Formal, standardized methods of assessment of family function have been developed and used successfully in the fields of family therapy and sociology (33,39,43,44). At least two methods of assessment have been described specifically for family practice (45,46). The method suggested below is neither formal nor standardized, but was developed from a combination of the above sources, Doherty and Baird (20), Minuchin (11,12,31), and the author's private practice experience with a family counselor. It is easily integrated into the routine history and physical exam (long or short version) and serves as a screening instrument. This method is similar to the use of the traditional review of systems already familiar to physicians. By utilizing this method, it becomes evident whether or not further assessment of the family system (more specific and formal) is needed.

During the initial consultation with a patient like the one above, the physician may explore the family dynamics and assess the relationship between the symptoms and the family system as part of the routine history and physical exam. This approach calls upon the *physician* to answer the questions from Table 3.3 by observing verbal and nonverbal responses of the patient (and families, if present) during the interview. This is a different process from just asking the questions directly of the patient. (Questions 1 and 2 may be asked and answered directly, *and* by observation.)

Question 1: Exactly what Happens Regarding the Symptoms and the Family?

This question is intended to ascertain the exact sequence of events with respect to the onset of symptoms. The goal is to track this sequence and note any response by and/or involvement with the family. (Who called the doctor? Who got upset, if anyone? How did the family respond to the illness? What were the associated events?). A second goal is to note any pattern or repeated sequence of events (see the pattern of Mr. Britt and his family below). One technique for tracking symptoms is to ask "sys-

TABLE 3.3. Four areas to explore in a family systems approach.

Tracking	Exactly what happens regarding the symptom and the family?	Note behaviors and responses of family members as they recall and explain the history. Track the exact sequence of events and symptoms.
Distress	What are the sources of distress for this patient? For this family?	Note emotionally sensitive issues for patient and family. What is the family heritage (regarding previous generations) with similar problems? Sketch a genogram. (Please see Chapter 8, Using the Genogram Clinically.)
Cohesiveness	How cohesive is this family? Is it more enmeshed or disengaged?	Note how involved the family is in the illness. Note how family members relate and communicate (directly and clearly, or not).
Adaptability	How adaptable or rigid is this patient and the family system?	Note how long the pattern of events has been recurring and how receptive the family is to a different opinion. Note how they respond to a suggestion for change (homework or task assignments).

What happened? Then what? And then what? What were you doing: sitting, standing, talking? What were you feeling? Then what happened? How did your family react? Who reacted the most? The least? The symptom can be tracked from onset to the present (or resolution, if not occurring now), noting any involvement with family members. The key is to encourage the patient to be specific ("What do you mean by a little while?" "What do you mean by 'nothing unusual?' " "What exactly were you eating, talking about, thinking about?").

When Mr. Britt was tracked through his symptoms, a pattern emerged:

1. Mr. Britt's employer would send him out of town on a business trip.
2. Mr. Britt called home after a few days "to check in" or Mrs. Britt might call him "to check on me."
3. After the telephone conversation Mr. Britt began to "feel lonely" and would find a local bar and begin to drink heavily.
4. After becoming drunk, he would call home and say, "Well, I did it again."
5. Mrs. Britt gathered the children (ages 16 and 22) and went to wherever he was staying and brought him home.
6. Mrs. Britt and their 16-year-old daughter nursed him back to health while he stayed home from work. The son and he did not speak. He felt he had "let down" his son and thought that his son was angry.

7. Mr. Britt felt guilty for a few days until either he apologized to all family members or enough time passed (a week or so) that he felt less guilty. He then returned to work and family members returned to their routine.

With little variation this cycle had occurred three to six times per year for 4 years. However, it seemed to be happening more often over the past year. Mr. Britt confirmed that he never desired to drink any alcohol while living at home (even if he had to travel out of town during the day).

Question 2: What Are the Sources of Distress for This Patient? For This Family?

The search for sources of distress may be structured by using the framework of the family life cycle (see Chapter 4, Table 4.2). The questions stem from the predictable issues and crises of this life cycle. Additional questions concerning unpredictable life events (loss of family member, job, divorce, disability, etc.) are asked to complement the life cycle issue.

Questions exploring sources of distress are: Have you thought about your children leaving home soon? How will that change things in your life? Do you and Mrs. Britt have much time together? Have you two discussed how things will change once they leave? What do you see as significant sources of distress in your life? How is your job? Do you like it? What is the worst thing about it? The best? What is going to happen if these symptoms continue? Is there anyone in the family background with a similar problem? How are they doing?

Although Mr. Britt discounted any sources of distress ("just the usual"), he worried about his absence from work due to sick leave, and he was concerned that his drinking was hurting the family. He was afraid that he might become an alcoholic, develop ulcers, lose his job, and/or see his family relationships deteriorate. At a later visit by both Mr. and Mrs. Britt, she expressed the concern that Mr. Britt was just like her father (an alcoholic).

When evaluating the role of distress in an illness, the emphasis is not upon how many (or how few) items a patient can list as potential sources of distress. The emphasis is upon how *much* distress this patient perceives *at this time; what* events are perceived as distressing; and *why* they are perceived so. Sometimes a patient feels little overt distress over many apparently stressful events; other times, a patient may feel very distressed over a single event (that may not seem significant to the physician). Distress is often not well identified within the individual's conscious awareness, and may be expressed through somatic symptoms (somatized) or disproportionate concern with minor symptoms. Physicians may gently uncover such covert distress and its relationship to the symptoms by simple inquiry. Distress is a personal and subjective state (although its effects can be objectively measured) and is best defined by the person experiencing it.

One other tool, the genogram, has proved useful in identifying factors influencing both patient and/or family. The genogram can be skillfully employed as a succinct sketch of the family heritage. It may reveal secrets and fears that constitute the family backdrop against which the present symptoms and events are interpreted (or misinterpreted) (18,19,46). In the Britt case, it was only while sketching the family tree that Mrs. Britt revealed that her father was an alcoholic. Her expression of previously unvoiced fears concerning Mr. Britt's pattern, and her description of her mother's "faithful" rescues, supplied information that was essential for understanding the present pattern and designing a plan to alter it.

During the initial interview, one can postulate likely sources of distress for the Britt family on the basis of the patient's history and knowledge of the family life cycle and family dynamics. At this point the following hypotheses were formulated:

1. The Britt family was locked into a dysfunctional cycle of events that was unsatisfactory for some or all members.
2. One of the Britt children resented having to rescue Mr. Britt.
3. Mrs. Britt, on the other hand, derived benefits from rescuing Mr. Britt (enjoying the fulfillment of her idea of a good wife by being the responsible one in the family).
4. The impending leaving of the children (ages 16 and 22) was a serious unexpressed concern of both Mr. and Mrs. Britt.
5. Mrs. Britt's family background contained a blueprint on which the present family structure and pattern fit (symptomatic drinking and rescues).

Question 3: How Cohesive is This Family System? Is It More Enmeshed or Disengaged?

It is important to know whether the Britt family system is enmeshed (overinvolved in one another's lives) or disengaged (underinvolved or cut off from each other), because an enmeshed family system may produce or maintain psychosomatic symptoms. On the other hand, a disengaged family system may limit or not provide mutual support and understanding, thus compromising the system's ability to adapt (6,19,28,30). Both types of systems may be perceived as tense and distressing by a family member, thus raising the frustration level of the patient or other members and raising the risk for illness (5,7,11,12,21,28,31,34,42).

It is difficult to accurately assess the cohesiveness of a family without seeing the entire family at one time and observing their interaction. It is useful, though, to form a hypothesis on the basis of the initial interview with the symptomatic member. Such a hypothesis may be confirmed, broadened, or rejected after further interactions between physician and family (separate office visits, hospital visits, family conference, home visits, and so on).

Questions exploring enmeshment are: How have these symptoms affected your roles in the family? How have they affected your spouse?

How do your children respond to your symptoms? What does your family think is the problem? These questions explore the interrelationship between symptoms (or illness) and the family. Another complementary task is to make observations about cohesion on the basis of Question 1 (what happens?) How involved was the Britt family, for example, in this whole sequence of events? As Mr. Britt tells his story, what are the family reactions (totally absorbed, bored, angry, afraid)?

When Mr. Britt was asked these questions, he expressed feelings of guilt concerning people filling in for him at home and work when he had been drinking. It was obvious that the family was involved in his drinking cycles as supportive rescuers. He saw himself as a frustrated, helpless victim. The drinking cycle of events had become part of the family's expected routine. "I can't go out of town. My mother may need me to help bail out my father." Mrs. Britt, however, was described as the strong one and Mr. Britt as the one with a problem. During the crisis, the son often moved into the father and husband roles. Mr. Britt's feeling that he should apologize to his son was somewhat of a role reversal, indicating that the generational boundaries were not clear nor well maintained.

For these reasons it was hypothesized that the Britt family was enmeshed. This was confirmed when, during a later visit, Mr. and Mrs. Britt repeatedly spoke for each other. A question to one would bring a response from the other, "Oh, he doesn't feel that way, Doctor. He feels . . ." Both Mr. and Mrs. Britt used the pronoun "we" frequently and seldom used "I." "We think (or feel) this way . . . ."

Also, Mr. and Mrs. Britt seldom spoke directly to each other, but rather triangled their communication constantly, a second feature of an enmeshed system. They talked *about* the drinking, *about* the children, or *about* each other ("I don't know why he does that.") but not about themselves and their relationship. Physicians often support or even demand this triangle by maintaining the discussion of physical symptoms. When family members are specifically asked to talk about themselves or to each other ("Why don't you ask her about that right now?"), the clinician can observe whether or not such a request raises anxiety, is followed, or is lost in the discussion of symptoms. Other features of Mr. and Mrs. Britt's interaction that typify enmeshed families are the interrupting, correcting, and rephrasing of Mr. Britt's responses "to make sure he is not misunderstood." Enmeshed families frequently describe themselves as "real close" and "never having a cross word," as both Mr. and Mrs. Britt did.

Question 4: How Adaptable or Rigid Is This Patient and the Family System?

A living system must be able to adapt to survive. If a system is too rigid, its members will experience more and more distress as the system is challenged by changes (illness, loss of member, etc.). A family system may have developed only one pattern to handle stressful life events. ("Mom can solve it; she'll know what to do."). Then, if their pattern is interrupted

(Mom gets sick) or overwhelmed (too many problems for Mom to solve), the family may become dysfunctional unless it can develop alternative patterns to manage stressful events (10,40,43,43,44).

One may hypothesize about the family's adaptability from the initial interview with the identified patient. In subsequent visits in the office, the hospital, or the home, this hypothesis may be tested by contact with individual members or the entire family. Questions that may help evaluate adaptability are similar to those for cohesiveness, with an emphasis on how entrenched the patterns are. Questions that help assess adaptability are: Who covers for you when you cannot parent or work? Is this the usual case? What would happen if they could not or did not cover for you? What is your daily routine with respect to work and family? How has it changed with your symptoms?

Again, the best way to assess adaptability of the system is by direct observation and/or by suggesting an alternative pattern (''Mrs. Britt, what would happen if you could not go get Mr. Britt?''), and noting response (''Oh, I could never do that, Doctor.'') In general, the longer and more frequently a pattern is repeated, the more entrenched or rigid it becomes (5,20).

The Britt family seemed fairly rigid because the cycle of events had been repeated regularly for 4 to 5 years. Mrs. Britt felt very comfortable in the rescuer role. Mr. Britt had accepted the sick role, although he seemed to be expressing desire for a change. The rest of the family co-operated willingly in the system, even though the son apparently harbored some unvocalized resentment of the cycle of events.

Directing the interview with this series of questions enabled the physician to identify an accurate sequence of events, family response patterns, family involvement, and rigidity of the Britt family system. Mr. Britt's family was clearly involved in the sequence of events surrounding his symptoms; they were unknowingly supporting and promoting his repeated cycle of symptoms (Question 1—tracking and pattern of events). The family and work systems were significant sources of distress for Mr. Britt. Mrs. Britt and her daughter appeared minimally distressed, and, in fact, derived satisfaction from the role of rescuer and caretaker. Mr. Britt's son seemed somewhat annoyed by the pattern (Question 2—distress). The Britt family system was enmeshed, with Mr. Britt lacking (by choice perhaps) autonomy, and caught in unresolved conflicts with Mrs. Britt (Questions 3—cohesiveness). The Britt family system appeared quite set (rigid) in the present pattern of events, demonstrating little adaptability (Question 4—adaptability).

Summary Points Concerning Clinical Example #2

In addition to selecting the partially accurate diagnostic labels of esophagitis and gastritis, the physician now understood a lot about how the family dynamics appear to be contributing significantly to the production and/or maintenance of these symptoms. The relationship between present symptoms and the family heritage for producing and/or dealing with such issues was productively explored. This family paradoxically criticized and supported the symptomatic drinking behavior. At the same time they avoided conflict and issues of impending life cycle changes. They used pseudocloseness to solve problems, and managed to maintain a tense, intact family system. The impending departure of the children was raising the intensity so that the system would be forced to change.

Physicians may hesitate to explore such issues, despite a strong clinical suspicion that the illness is complicated by such factors. Clinicians frequently feel they must first prove there is no physical problem before addressing obvious psychological factors. Such strict division of factors fails to recognize the relationship between what people believe and feel and how they act (resultant symptoms) (5,13,25,27,37,47–49). In this case the significance of the family system as a contributing factor was evaluated by asking probing questions and making informed observations. Mr. Britt's family system was *initially* considered as a potential source of the symptoms instead of being considered only after repeated laboratory tests and X-rays. Further diagnostic work-up may indeed reveal a peptic ulcer as an additional explanation of his symptoms. This does not negate the influence of psychosocial factors. From the first encounter the physician was able to say, "Mr. Britt, I would like you to have some tests to clarify what is going on in your stomach. But whether you have an ulcer or not, there are several stress-related issues that I think are important for us to address. I recommend we start on these while we pursue further testing." This approach bypassed the resistance that might have been forthcoming should the physician adopt a rule-out-organic-disease-first approach. Patients may feel rejected or insulted with an approach that implies they have psychological or stress-related problems because all the tests are negative (3,7,18,19,20).

Mr. Britt was offered the usual medical regimen, and the physician further suggested that he and Mrs. Britt return for a follow-up visit to further further discuss related issues with both of them. A management plan that failed to recognize the family system and the possibility of preventing his drinking binges would have treated his symptoms without dealing with other important factors. Another management option for the physician is to consult and/or work with a family therapist to deal with the family aspect of the illness (19). By utilizing the principles of family systems theory, the physician arrived at a more complete diagnosis and understanding of the illness (rather than just a diagnostic label), so that a more thorough and specific management plan was designed.

Indications for Exploring the Family System

Exploring these four areas is suggested as a valuable part of the routine history and physical (see Table 3.2). The intensity and thoroughness of exploration is guided by the responses and situation (school physical, acute illness, repeated symptoms). In several clinical situations a more detailed approach will be particularly productive and time saving in the long run (16,20,50,51).

Serious (Especially Terminal) Illness

The family always experiences a heavy impact when one member is seriously or terminally ill (23). The hospital (or home) may be a natural and convenient place to address issues raised by the illness of one member (1,20,23,48). In addition, chemical abuse or dependence generally involves the family as both resource for and resistance to improvement (20,22,52).

Parent–Child Relationship Problems

Children may act out the chaos or conflict in the parental subsystem (29,30,53). This is a natural entry point to discuss the effects of the acting out on the family and the spouses (or single parent), and the plan for management (20,29,30,53).

Psychosomatic Symptoms or Psychophysiologic Illness

Ample evidence indicates that psychosocial distress either produces or complicates many illnesses, such as peptic ulcer disease, migraine headaches, tension headaches, irritable bowel syndrome, and ulcerative colitis (Table 3.2). Without exploring the stress-related factors for such symptoms, an inordinate amount of time may be spent treating and discussing the same symptoms repeatedly. A systems approach may enlighten both patient and physician and provide a more effective method of management (2,6,14,17,20,21,27,37,47).

Sexual Dysfunction

Some symptoms of sexual dysfunction are the result of misinformation and basic misunderstanding. Family physicians, by their willingness to discuss such issues, may legitimize an open exchange about such topics, and thus discover that a simple explanation or recommended resource will resolve the problem (2,54). Using a systems approach (see Table 3.2) to addressing the relationship uncovers significant issues for physician and patient while sidestepping the trap of assigning blame (20).

Family Life Cycle Tasks and Issues

As described in detail in Chapter 4, the family life cycle tasks and predictable crises are high risk periods for family distress and thus for illness and consultation with the physician (4,8,16,17).

Problems in Practice

"Good" or "Bad" Family

There is a tendency to approach family systems with an attitude of "It's either a bad family or a good family." The terms bad and good are best avoided because they are so relative and vague that they generate more confusion than clarity (and prompt defensiveness from the families who do not like their label). Such labeling also interferes with the clinician's ability to accurately assess symptoms and family patterns. Physicians may begin to dread or chide families with a "bad" label, thus reinforcing the system and becoming dysfunctionally entangled (see below). The systems view is not to expose a family as unhealthy but to help a clinician understand why this family member has this illness at this time, and what factors in the family system, if any, are contributing to, affected by, or complicating the illness (7,22,31,32).

Area Overlap

Admittedly the questions and observations used to evaluate the Britt family overlap. When searching for a pattern of events, for example, one may observe enmeshment, or note rigidity. With practice the principles are integrated into the diagnostic process, so that the questions become a natural part of the interview, and the observations are absorbed simultaneously.

Systems Change

Family systems change depending upon membership, conditions, and other influences (41). A disorganized system may suddenly organize with the appearance (or disappearance) of one member. A system that is rigidly enmeshed while in crisis may be quite flexible or even disengaged once the crisis passes (1,31). Such changes in family system may affect the physician's understanding and management of symptms.

Family Resistance

Patients and families may resist accepting or even considering the possibility that the family is contributing to the problem. The patient may insist upon discussing physical symptoms only. Denial is not unique to family systems problems, though. Patients also sometimes deny that they have heart trouble or high blood pressure or emphysema. An effective process for managing resistance in the initial interview is straightforward, empathetic, and firm, e.g., "Mr. Britt, I understand that you don't see the point of discussing some of these issues. But, I think discussing these issues will give me a better understanding of your symptoms and I would like to pursue them. Now, I need some information about your job."

Physician's Family Heritage

As previously mentioned, the physician has his/her own set of beliefs and emotional connections derived from his/her own family background (see "Understanding Family Systems Helps Avoid Entanglement," above). Physicians may be frustrated and paralyzed by certain families or family members. Beginning to understand how their own families work will enable physicians to recognize their own vulnerabilities with certain types of families. They may function more effectively and with greater satisfaction as a result (18–20).

Summary

Factors that seem critical to the understanding and management of illness are not adequately addressed in many textbook descriptions. An approach that isolates symptoms and individuals from the context in which they occur frequently lacks the breadth and accuracy needed for effective management. The family system forms a portion of the context that influences the health and illness of its members. Family systems theories offer a framework that helps explain confusing symptoms, behaviors, and difficulties of patients, doctors, and families. While there is no one universally accepted family theory, physicians may find in the principles discussed here a conceptual nidus around which vague clinical suspicions may crystallize. Although learning and applying skills for working with family systems requires time and effort, family-oriented medical care is more effective than the isolated individual approach. It also proves in the long run to be more accurate and more satisfying for the doctor, the patient, and the family because it offers a framework for understanding symptoms in the contexts in which they occur, individual and family. Instead of rigidly and independently prescribing a management schema *for* the patient, a family systems orientation means working *with* patients and families to design a strategy that addresses symptoms within the context of their lives.

References

1. Satir V: Conjoint Family Therapy. Palo Alto, CA, Science and Behavior Books, 1967.
2. Balint M: The Doctor, His Patient and the Illness. London, Pittman Medical Publishing Company, 1957.
3. Rakel RE: Preventive medicine in practice, in Principles of Family Medicine. Philadelphia, Saunders, 1977.
4. Huygen FJA: Family Medicine: the Medical Life History of Families. New York, Brunner/Mazel, 1982.
5. Bowen M: The use of family theory in clinical practice. Comprehensive Psychiatry 1966:7:345–374.

6. Brody H: The systems view of man: Implications for medicine, science, and ethics. Perspect Biol Med 1973;17(Autumn):71–92.

7. Hadley TR, Jacob T, Milliones J, Caplan J, Spitz D: The relationship between family developmental crises and the appearance of symptoms in a family member. Fam Process 1974;13:207–214.

8. Holmes TH, Rahe RH: The social readjustment rating scale. Psychosom Med 1967;11:213–218.

9. Jackson DD: Family homeostasis and the physician. Calif Med 1965;104(4):239–242.

10. Meissner WW: Family dynamics and psychosomatic process. Fam Process 1966;5:142–161.

11. Minuchin S: Psychosomatic Families. Cambridge, MA, Harvard University Press, 1978.

13. Minuchin S, Baker L, Rosman BL, Liebman R, Milman L, Todd TC: A conceptual model of psychosomatic illness in children. Arch Gen Psychiatry 1975;32:1031–1038.

14. Bursten B: Family dynamics and illness behavior. Gen Pract 1964;29(5):142–145.

15. Christie-Seely J: Teaching the family system concept in family medicine. J Fam Pract 1981;13:391–40.

16. Christie-Seely J: Preventive medicine and the family. Can Fam Phys 1983;29:533–540.

17. Christie-Seely J: Life stress and illness: A systems approach. Can Fam Phys 1983;29:533–540.

18. Crouch MA: Working with one's own family: Another path for professional development. Fam Med 1986;18:93–98.

19. Crouch MA, Davis TC: Working with families: I. Basic family oriented health care, in Robertson D (ed): Textbook of Family Medicine Chicago, Yearbook Medical Publisher (in press).

20. Doherty WJ, Baird MA: Family Therapy and Family Medicine. New York, Guilford Press, 1983.

21. Ackerman SH, Manaker S, Cohen MI: Recent separation and the onset of peptic ulcer disease in older children and adolescents. Psychosom Med 1981;43:305–310.

22. Cleveland M: Families and adolescent drug abuse: Structures analysis of children's roles. Fam Process 1981;20:394–404.

23. Fisher JV, Barnett BL, Collins J: The post suicide family and the family physician. J Fam Pract 1976;3:263–267.

24. Medalie JH: Family Medicine—Principles and Applications. Baltimore, Williams & Wilkins, 1978.

25. Mechanic D: The influence of mothers on their children's health attitudes and behavior. Pediatrics 1964;33:444–453.

26. Ransom D, Vandervoort HE: The development of family medicine. JAMA 1973;225:1098–1102.

27. Engel GL: The clinical application of the biopsychosocial model. Am J Psychiatry 1980;137:535–544.

28. Lewis JM: The family and physical illness. Texas Med 1976;72:43–49.

29. Liebman R, Minuchin S, Baker L: The use of structural family therapy in the treatment of intractable asthma. Am J Psychiatry 1974;131:535–540.

30. Liebman R, Minuchin S, Baker L: The role of the family in the treatment of anorexia nervosa. Child Psychiatry 1974;13:264–274.

31. Minuchin S: Families and Family Therapy. Cambridge, MA, Harvard University Press, 1974.
32. Barnhill L.R. Healthy family systems. Fam Coordinator 1979;28(1):94–100.
33. Epstein NB, Bishop DS, Levin S: The McMaster model of family functioning. J Marriage Fam Counsel 1978;4(4):19–31.
34. Marshall JR, Neill J: The removal of a psychosomatic symptom and effects on the marriage. Fam Process 16:273–280.
35. Meyer RJ, Haggerty RJ: Streptococcal infection in families. Pediatrics 1962;29:539–549.
36. Quill TE: Somatization disorder. JAMA 1985;254:3075–3079.
37. Steinglass P: A life history model of the alcoholic family. Fam Process 1980;19:214–226.
38. Jackson DD: The study of the family. Fam Process 1965;4:1–20.
39. Olsen DH, Sprenkle DH, Russell CS: Circumplex model of marital and family systems: I. Cohesion and adaptability dimensions, family types, and clinical applications. Fam Process 1979;18:3–28.
40. Jackson DD: Family rules: Marital quid pro quo. Arch Gen Psychiatry 1965;12:589–594.
41. Walsh F (ed): Normal Family Processes. New York, Guilford Press, 1982.
42. Livsey CG: Physical illness and family dynamics. Adv Psychosom Med 1972;8:237–251.
43. Russell CS: Circumplex model of marital and family systems: III. Empirical evaluation with families. Fam Process 1979;18:29–45.
44. Sprenkle DH, Olsen DH: Circumplex model of marital systems: An empirical study of clinical and non-clinic couples. J Marriage Fam Counsel 1978;4(2):59–74.
45. Arbogast RC, Scratton JM, Krick JP: The family as a patient: Preliminary experiences with a recorded assessment schema. J Fam Pract 1978;7:1151–1157.
46. Jolly W, Froom J, Rosen MG: The genogram. J Fam Pract 1980;10:251–255.
47. Engel GL: The need for a new medical model: A challenge for biomedicine. Science 1977;196:129–136.
48. Parkes CM: Effects of bereavement on physical and mental health, a study of the medical records of widows. Br Med J 1964;2:274–279.
49. Widmer RB, Cadoret RJ, North CS: Depression in family practice: Some effects on spouses and children. J Fam Pract 1980;10:45–51.
50. Schmidt DD: When is it helpful to convene the family? J Fam Pract 1983;16:967–973.
51. Smilkstein G. The family in trouble—How to tell. J Fam Pract 1975;2:19–24.
52. Stanton MD: The family and drug abuse: Concepts and rationale, in Bratter TE, Forrest GG (eds) Alcoholism and Substance Abuse: Strategies for Clinical Intervention. New York, Free Press, 1985, pp 398–429.
53. Pfeffer CR: The family system of suicidal children. Am J Psychother 1981;35:330–341.
54. Kaplan HS: The New Sex Therapy. New York, Brunner/Mazel, 1974.
55. Schmidt DD: Family determinates of disease: Depressed lymphocyte function following the loss of a spouse. Fam Syst Med 1983;1(1):33–39.
56. Medalie JH, Snyder M, Groen JJ, et al: Angina pectoris among 10,000 men; 5-year incidence and univariate analysis. Am J Med 1973;55:583–594.

CHAPTER 4

The Family Life Cycle in Medical Practice

Leonard Roberts

One of the most useful frameworks for viewing the family as a discrete system (rather than just a collection of individuals) is the family life cycle. Emerging from the observations of sociologists (1–6), psychiatrists (7), and family therapists (8–9), the family life cycle is a logical extension of its clinical predecessors, child (10) and adult (11–14) growth and development. Individual growth and development do not stop at age 21, nor do they take place in a vacuum. Different individual stages of development occur simultaneously in different family members—the onset of adolescence in a child and midlife crisis in a parent, for instance. The concept of the family life cycle has been applied clinically in family therapy (8,9) and family practice (15–17). This chapter will define the family life cycle, illustrate how it can be a useful adjunct in medical practice, and discuss its logistical and theoretical limitations for such practice.

The family life cycle divides the life history of a family into observable, predictable stages of development. Each stage is characterized by (a) developmental tasks pertinent to that stage, and (b) predictable crises associated with the accomplishment (or nonaccomplishment) of those tasks (2). Table 4.1 lists one version of the family life cycle stages, the chronological ages that roughly correlate with each stage, and the comparable individual adult developmental stages (2,11–14). The developmental tasks of each stage are given in Table 4.2.

It should be kept in mind that the families from which these observations were drawn were most frequently middle class, American, caucasian, and living in the era 1940–1970. Clinicians deal with all types of families that may differ significantly from the characteristics of this population. In fact, the "traditional family" of two adults, two children, and only one parent employed constitutes only 11–13% of our population (2,3,5). Blended or remarried families, other ethnic groups, single-parent families, families without children, families at the extremes of the socioeconomic scale, and so forth continue to be studied, and more specific observations are being made (2,3,5,18–20). Still, Duvall's (2) family life cycle is useful as a skeletal framework as long as these limitations are kept in mind.

TABLE 4.1. Comparison of family life cycle stages with simultaneous individual life cycle stages by age.*

Family life cycle stages	Age	Individual adult life cycle stages
	18	
I. Family formation		Early adult transition
	20	
	25	Early adulthood
II. Childbearing families (oldest child 0–30 months)		
	30	Age 30 transition
III. Family with preschool-age children (oldest child 2½–6)	35	
		Young adult life "settling down"
IV. Family with school-age children (oldest child 6–13)	40	
		Mid-life transition
V. Family with teenage children (oldest child 13–18)	45	
	50	
VI. Family dispersion (oldest child 18+)	55	Mid-adult life
VII. Older couple or couple again	60	
		Late adulthood
	65+	

*Modified from: Duvall EM: Marriage and Family Development, ed 5. Philadelphia, Lippincott, 1977; Sheehy, G: Passages. New York, Dutton, 1976; and Levinson, D: The Seasons of a Man's Life. New York, Knopf, 1978.

In the text that follows, after each stage is described there are examples demonstrating the relevance to and application in medical practice. The objective, with respect to each example, is to answer each of the following questions: (a) At what stage of development is this patient and his/her family? (b) What are the developmental tasks and crises of that stage? (c) How does this information fit with the patient's expressed reason for coming to the physician?

Stage I—Family Formation

The new family begins when two people leave their respective families of origin and decide to live together as a couple. The three tasks that characterize this event are: (a) establishing the couple bond; (b) adjusting

TABLE 4.2. Family life cycle stages and developmental tasks.*

Life cycle stage	Developmental tasks
I—Family formation	1. Developing autonomy. 2. Adjustment to new role and new person. 3. Establishment of couple bond.
II—Childbearing families	1. Adaptation to new person. 2. Adaptation to new role (parenthood). 3. Maintaining couple bond.
III—Families with preschool-age children	1. Making room for new self (individuation of child). 2. Making room for sexuality (sexual identity of child). 3. Coping with inadequate energy and privacy (by the couple).
IV—Families with school-age children	1. Establishing new boundaries. 2. Establishing new responsibilities.
V—Families with teenagers	1. Expanding boundaries. 2. Expanding responsibilities. 3. Preparing for the leaving of children.
VI—Family dispersion	1. Departure of first child (and each child respectively). 2. Renegotiating the couple bond.
VII—Older couple (or couple again)	1. Facing retirement. 2. Facing aging (health limits). 3. Redefining couple bond.

*Modified from: Duvall EM: Marriage and Family Development, ed 5. Philadelphia, Lippincott, 1977.

to the new partner and role; and (c) becoming independent of one's family of origin.

These seem fairly straightforward, but are achieved only with difficulty, because the tasks may be complex (2,3,8,12). First of all, autonomy is a matter of degree, i.e., is this person autonomous enough to establish the new couple relationship, and to leave the family of origin? The goal is not to become completely free of the family of origin, since such complete freedom also would sever the support from and the responsibility to the family of origin. Minuchin described a balance between enmeshment (little or no individual autonomy) and disengagement (complete cutoff) as the functional optimum (21). Bowen described individuation from an undifferentiated familial mass (22,23). Developing autonomy is a process that requires years (and mistakes) to realize. It is difficult for most people in our culture to functionally separate before age 30, especially if one lives geographically close to one's family of origin and/or is financially dependent on parents or other relatives (22–24).

The process of adjusting to a new partner and a new role is simultaneous and sometimes identical with the process of forming a bond, or contract, between two people. The nature of this bond is very important to the new family, because it sets the tone for how differences will be handled, how disagreements are to be negotiated, when and how the family will eat, play, work, spend money, express emotions, express sexuality, go to the doctor, visit in-laws—i.e., how the family will live and function (8,21,24) Predictable crises arise from the difficulty of achieving autonomy from one's family of origin and in adjusting to a new role.

Clinical Example #1: Family Formation

Mr. Smith, a 28-year-old white male, presented to his physician with a chief complaint of "upset stomach" and "nervousness" that had been occurring for 6–8 weeks. The upset stomach was described as "stomach pain," abdominal discomfort, but not really painful, although occasionally he got a "crampy" sensation across his abdomen. He had had intermittent constipation over the past month, but had no other gastrointestinal symptoms. His nervousness occurred the past 8–10 weeks, and was worse the past 2 weeks. He described this as a generally uneasy feeling, with occasional spells of being very upset for no apparent reason. He experienced early morning awakening and had difficulty getting to sleep some evenings. He had not lost weight.

Mr. Smith had been in generally good health with no hospital admissions and no visits to the physician except for "job physicals." A review of symptoms was negative.

Mr. and Mrs. Smith had been married for 6 months and had no children. When asked how married life was going, he said "Fine." Both sets of parents were living and in good health. There was no history of major illness in either family. Both Mr. and Mrs. Smith were the only children of their respective families. He stated that his wife visits her mother often, and that they ate Sunday dinner every weekend with at least one set of parents.

Except for signs of anxiety (tense facial muscles and a worried look on his face) and minimal epigastric discomfort to palpation, the physical examination was normal. A brief mental status exam was unremarkable. When asked if he felt "down", Mr. Smith said he felt a "little depressed" and tired. He denied suicidal ideation.

The patient's nuclear family is clearly in Stage I of the family life cycle. His family of origin, however, is in Stage VI and he's still part of that family too. The developmental tasks (and the predictable crises) of these stages are listed in Table 4.2. To unravel how this connects with the patient's chief complaint, it is useful to consider how symptoms are thought to arise.

According to the biopsychosocial model, for illness or symptoms to occur there are at least three requirements (25–27). The first of these is physiologic vulnerability. Predisposition to producing excessive acid in the stomach, to muscle tension, to bronchospasm, and so forth are examples of this background vulnerability. These preexisting pathophysiologic conditions are not necessarily caused by the stress-related factors, but are influenced by them—e.g., diabetes, *Herpes simplex* virus types I and II, arthritis, psoriasis, and numerous other chronic illnesses (26,28–31).

A second requirement for illness to occur is a stressful event or challenge to the system (exposure e to contagious organism, loss of a family member, etc.). Stressors may be biological, psychosocial, or environmental, and changes that appear to the observer to be positive (a job promotion, for example) may be more stressful to the individual than other apparently negative events (8,24,30).

Compromise of one or more physiologic systems (immune, nervous, cardiovascular, etc.) is the third factor illness requires. A compromise that is sufficiently severe, occurring in conjunction with matching physiologic vulnerability or preexisting pathophysiology, can result in such problems as symptomatic infection, coronary artery occlusion, or "nervous breakdown" (see Chapter 5 on "Families and Illness"). Stress occurring in the absence of a suitable vulnerability or pathophysiology, or stress that does not critically compromise any body systems, may increase an individual's anxiety and impair general functioning without precipitating clinical illness (8,24,26,30).

In Mr. Smith's case, his ability to adapt was overwhelmed by the changes that had taken place (marriage plus the continued stresses he felt from his family of origin). As a result, his digestion worsened, his eating habits became more haphazard, his sleep became more disturbed, his frustration increased—in short, he became sick.

There is a tendency on the part of physicians to identify stress-related symptoms as either real or not real, organic or functional. Mr. Smith's illness was real to him—real pain, real fatigue, real indigestion, and real frustration. The illness occurred as a combination of the presence of distressing events and his temporary inability to cope. The absence of either would allow him to get better. Improving his defenses against illness with antacids, better eating habits, and/or coping skills would help restore his health. Both vulnerability and stress must be present for illness to occur, and therapy may be directed at either or both.

Mr. Smith's symptoms and illness were affected by the predictable frustration of having difficulty with developmental tasks of the life cycle. Knowing the background life cycle information sensitizes the clinician to the age-appropriate issues of autonomy, adjustment, and establishment of a couple bond. The distress that often accompanies these tasks is thereby recognized, and the physician understands the patient and his/her chief complaint more accurately. To discern issues such as autonomy and to assess the distress that may accompany them, the clinician may utilize systemic questions (26,32,33) (see Chapter 3). The physician asked Mr. Smith a number of questions about issues of autonomy: How do you feel about seeing parents (yours or hers) every Sunday? What time do you have for yourself/or for fun? How has it been to leave home? Do you feel like you have "fully" left? Do you ever feel like going back home? Do you ever feel pulled back home? How did your parents feel about your leaving? Your marriage?

Questions were also asked about the couple bond and adjustment. How did it come about that every Sunday you visit one set of parents or the other? How satisfactory is it now? How do you and Mrs. Smith decide these things? How do you know when she disagrees? How has all this affected your sex life? (Asking "How's the marriage?" almost always receives the reflex response "Fine.") How much time do you have together free from other duties and obligations? What has been the best thing about marriage? The worst? Unexpected things?

Each interviewer develops his/her own style and set of questions. A direct, brief series of questions such as those above can enlighten both physician and patient. These questions offered Mr. Smith an opportunity to express any hidden agenda items that do not carry an organic label and thus are not perceived as legitimate for discussion. They also enable the clinician to assess the symptoms in terms of the family life cycle, the family system, and the amount of distress the patient feels in that system with respect to the stage-related tasks and crises. In Mr. Smith's case, for instance, further exploration of issues revealed that he was feeling quite torn between attending to his own family (being a son), his wife (being a husband), and her family (being an in-law), and wanting more time alone (being an individual). These roles encompass basic autonomy and couple-bond issues.

Another benefit of exploring the family life cycle is that it gives the physician a more complete history of the Smith family. In addition to knowing whether members of a family had medical diagnoses (diabetes, hypertension, etc.), the physician knows something of the family function (or dysfunction), and the character of relationships. This information in Mr. Smith's case allowed the physician to assess to what degree family factors were contributing to his distress and/or how they might aid his relief. His roles as worker and provider had been compromised, and he felt worse just thinking about going over to his in-laws.

The physician was convinced of the significance of psychosocial factors in this case through positive data collection instead of the inadequate method of diagnosis by exclusion ("I can't find anything wrong with you, so it must be in your head."). Mr. Smith may very well have had a developing duodenal ulcer or any one of numerous organic causes for his symptoms. By using the family life cycle, however, it is easy to identify sources of distress that, in addition to the organic factors, needed addressing for optimal management. Consistent with this approach, the physician told Mr. Smith, "I don't know at this point if your abdominal discomfort is an ulcer, and we can do some testing to clarify that. However, whether you have an ulcer or not there are other stress-related issues that could produce or add to your symptoms, and I recommend that we begin to work on those, too."

In summary, Stage I (Family Formation) is characterized by the developmental tasks of achieving autonomy from the family of origin, adjusting to the new partner and role, and establishing a new couple bond. Predictably stressful crises arise in the attempt to achieve each of these tasks that may be clinically relevant for optimal management.

Stage II—Childbearing Families (First child 0–30 months)

Adults in childbearing families, often still only partially successful with family formation tasks, face the additional tasks of (a) adapting to a new person (new child), (b) adapting to a new role (parent), and (c) maintaining the couple bond (retaining an active spouse relationship).

Anytime another person moves into (or out of) a family system there are changes—new schedules, limits, and responsibilities that require a shift from the old system of doing things. The two-person marital dyad becomes a triad, inevitably developing triangular interactions with some degree of tension and conflict (8,22,24,29). The new person in this case, however, is an infant, requiring each spouse to move into a new role, that of parenting (nurturing, feeding, protecting, playing). The detailed functions of parenting must be learned, although role enactment is based on a blueprint drawn from the individual's genetic makeup and the respective families of origin. This blueprint will require modifications because each family differs from the families of origin, and because some of the preexisting patterns may not be conducive to optimal functioning of the new family (8,21,24).

Although some attenuation of the couple bond is to be expected due to the unavoidable drain on the time and energy of each parent (usually more so with the mother), the husband–wife bond remains crucial to family function (21). The advent of a new child and the subsequent constant changes in the expanded family require an active, if not conscious effort to maintain the spouse or couple bond. The long-term stability and viability of the family is jeopardized when the parent–child bonds are overly intense and the spousal bond critically weakened (8,21,24).

Strain on Husband–Wife Relationship

After the birth of the first child, the male partner may invest more time in work (the provider role), spending little time either in the husband role or in the father role. He may not actively parent—hold or play with the baby, change diapers, feed, bathe, or comfort the baby, and so forth. The disengaged father role describes this distancing, and it may be supported (and even encouraged) by the spouse. The new mother, on the other hand, may overinvest herself in the mother role, even though she may also be working outside the home. While this tendency is initially the natural course of events, some families get stuck in unbalanced and unsatisfactory role functions. There are no pat guidelines for evaluating role balance, and no right or wrong amount of time for each role in a given family. Problems arise when a dynamic system becomes static in some respects, creating a dysfunctional equilibrium. At this point the member feeling the most distress may present to the physician with fatigue, malaise, headaches, or any number of chief complaints (8,21,24,31). The physician may recommend an expensive laboratory evaluation or attempt symptomatic treatment that will probably prove unsatisfactory until these factors are addressed.

Potential problems may occur with prolongation of the disengaged father position. Active parenting is difficult from a disengaged position ("Who knows what he thinks? The children don't really know him. He's no help with the children.") It is also difficult to be an active spouse from such a distance ("I never see him. I don't know if he really cares about me. We never talk anymore.") (8,21,24).

If the woman overdoes the mother role on a long-term basis to the exclusion of her other functions, there are some other risks to the family and individual integrity. The marital couple bond may be irretrievably weakened due to insufficient couple time and connectedness. The mother may shut the father out from an active parenting role to bolster her own sense of importance. When the children leave home, such a mother role will no longer be needed, and the mother may feel she has lost her central identity. This may be avoided if the woman who is heavily invested in the mother role can adjust to reclaim other roles (self, wife, daughter, and so forth) (8,21,24,33,34).

Family members must work out satisfactory ways to give and receive feedback and fulfill the roles of parent, spouse, worker, and individual self if they are to avoid getting stuck in an unsatisfactory system. Difficulty often arises in balancing roles because no two individuals agree completely on how much time to spend in each position, nor on what behaviors constitute fulfilling that role satisfactorily.

Child-focused Family

Another predictable dysfunctional equilibrium for the childbearing family involves a general overfocusing on the child (or children). One or more of the children becomes the central focus for most adult thought, emotions, actions, and planning. Child-centered activity and planning occur in all families, but if everything hinges upon constant parental monitoring of the children's happiness, the family will be dysfunctional to some extent (21,24,31). This places a great deal of pressure on the child(ren). In effect, the parents are saying "We live only for you, i.e., make us happy." Second, a child who seems to be the cement that binds a shaky relationship between two adults also becomes a wedge separating the spouses (14,23). Communications in dysfunctional families are often channeled (indirectly) through the child instead of being made directly from spouse to spouse.

Love, anger, requests, refusals, and differences are "triangled" through the child (21,24,31) (see Clinical Examples #2 and #3, below).

Unfinished Business

With each stage from this point on, leftover or unresolved issues from earlier stages commonly generate crises. There is a general overlapping and continuum as families move from one stage to the next. Successful negotiation of tasks hinges upon resolution of prior issues. It is more difficult to become an effective parent, for instance, if one has not severed enough ties from the family of origin (autonomy) (8,21,24). The passage of time forces more issues upon the family regardless of whether the family has completed the tasks of previous stages.

Clinical Example #2: Unfinished Business

Mrs. Jones, a 30-year-old woman in generally good health, presented with a chief complaint of headache, described as a "band around my head" occurring most days for the past 6 weeks, accompanied by occasional nausea but no vomiting. The longest duration was 2–3 days consecutively, and the shortest duration was "off and on" for one day. There was no prodrome and no other neurological symptoms or sequelae. Aspirin had previously relieved the headache for several days to a week, but the past few months the headache recurred more frequently. Previous work-up 6 months ago included a normal brain scan, computerized tomography (CT) scan, lumbar puncture, and electroencephalogram. She was told that this was a tension headache and she needed to relax. Otherwise, Mrs. Jones was in generally good health, with no other medical problems. Mrs. Jones had been married for 6 years and her husband was a third-year student in medical school. She had two children, age 2½ years and 6 months, who "drive me nuts."

Both sets of parents were alive and in generally good health. They saw the husband's parents frequently, eating at his mother's house each weekend after he rounded at the hospital. The patient and her husband were both only children (no siblings). Except for the strained tone of her voice and an angry facial expression, the physical examination was normal. Neurological exam was completely within normal limits.

Considering the family life cycle issues in Stage II, it seemed appropriate to obtain more information about the patient's adaptation to the new role of parent, maintenance of the couple bond, and issues of unfinished business. Questions designed to elicit such information were asked. Who takes care of the children mostly—washing, feeding, diaper changes, playing, etc.? What happens when you have a headache? Who cares for the children then? How often do you get time off? How has it been to have two preschoolers? What do you miss the most since having children?

Specific couple bond questions were also asked. What did you two do together before you had children? When is your time together now? How do you two work out disagreements? How have these symptoms affected your spouse? Your sex life?

These questions revealed that Mrs. Jones was totally invested (and felt trapped) in the mother role and had lost touch with her roles as wife and individual. As previously mentioned, the mother's enmeshment with the new baby is typical initially for families with infants. Mrs. Jones felt stuck in the mother role, however, and wanted relief. In addition, she and Mr. Jones had some unfinished business from the family formation stage. Mrs. Jones expressed that Mr. Jones had spent more time in son and student roles than she expected or wanted. Since Mrs. Jones felt unable to discuss these frustrations and differences with her husband, she communicated her anger through the children and her headache. When she had a headache she could not effectively take care of and discipline the children, and she became angry with them quickly. The anger that might be more appropriately directed toward her husband was instead expressed in her inability to function as an effective mother, building frustration and finally producing a tension headache. Given this understanding of her symptoms, management included the usual medical recommendations and a suggestion that Mr. and Mrs. Jones come in together. At that office visit the physician offered to help them identify some of the stresses that were contributing to her headache. In the long run this would mean renegotiating the couple bond and each one redefining expectations of self and each other (2,8,15,16).

Physicians are rightfully concerned about the organic basis for symptoms. This concern, however, may result in clinical foot-dragging when it comes to identifying significant stress-related factors. Mrs. Jones might have had a brain tumor that was undetectable, or atypical migraines, or any of a number of other causes for headaches. These possibilities cannot be totally dismissed just because there was evidence of a relationship between the symptoms and family distress. The diagnosis of stress-related symptoms, however, was not based solely upon exclusion of organic diagnoses but on the positive findings in the history. Thorough physical examination and normal laboratory findings helped confirm the unlikelihood of other serious pathophysiology. In fact, even if Mrs. Jones were to have a brain tumor, there were still a number of stress-related issues that required attention for successful management of this case. While further work-up for organic causes might be advisable at some point, physician and patient had already begun work on the stress-related issues.

Reassurance requires more than simply telling a patient not to worry. Previously Mrs. Jones was told not to worry after her work-up. Although intended to reassure Mrs. Jones, such advice was interpreted as discounting her symptoms, rejecting her, implying she was a "crock," and at least lacking in empathy. If she were able to not worry at this point, she would not have arranged for another opinion. This "shotgun" reassurance approach failed to consider other sources related to her headaches. Reassurance is more effective when specific, i.e., when the clinician understands what is worrying the patient. In Mrs. Jones' case she was worried that the headache may be dangerous (brain tumor) and that if they were tension headaches, they would never stop. Taking a complete history (including family stressors) and a neurological examination proved reassuring to her. The physician's explanation of symptoms on positive findings in the history enhanced the relief. Instead of saying "you're under stress," the physician helped Mrs. Jones identify specific areas of distress and frustration, raising the probability of successful management of symptoms (8,21,24,32).

Stage III—Families with Preschoolers

The developmental tasks of Stage III are making room for new self (individuation of child), making room for sexuality (learning to be a boy or girl), and coping with the shortage of energy and privacy as parents. As the child grows and begins to walk, babble, and explore, there is a natural distancing and attenuation of the parent–child bond. The child expresses his/her own opinions—"No" or "By myself." A vital developmental stage for the child is learning that he/she is separate and different, and how to express this differentness (often called "the terrible two's"). For the family the task is that of learning to allow individuality while still maintaining the family functions of protection, nurture, and guidance (2,8,21,24).

The preschooler is also learning that he/she is either a boy or girl. The family influences the attitudes and behaviors that children formulate about sexuality, i.e., they learn what it means in their family to be a male or female. Do males leave in the morning and come home at night? Do females do the same or work differently? Do males yell at females, vice versa, or both? How do males express anger, sadness, and affection? How do females express strong feelings? Through thousands of interactions children unconsciously learn what it means to be a boy, a girl, a Mama, a Daddy (2,21,24).

Spouses may struggle to find adequate time or space for each other and for themselves individually. The demands upon time and energy by the children are potentially endless. The challenge of a new male or female in the family can be particularly difficult (little girls competing for Dad's attention, little boys for Mom's). What limits are appropriate? Who will set the limits, and how will they set them? Predictably, crises develop as small children place more demands on the system, in addition to the unresolved issues of earlier stages (2,8,21,24).

Clinical Example #3: Triangulated Bladder

Brent was a 4½-year-old child with a 6-month history of bedwetting. Brent was toilet trained by age 30 months, but in the last 6–8 months began bedwetting 1–2 nights per week. He was without evidence of infection and, otherwise, was without complaints. Mrs. Clark, Brent's mother, brought Brent in and seemed very upset, even tearful. She said she was afraid that something serious was wrong and that something must be done. Immunizations were up to date. Growth curves were maintained. Brent's parents had been married for 6 years and were both in good health. Brent was the older of two children. He has a 15-month-old sister, Jenny. Mrs. Clark did not work outside the home. Mr. Clark was self-employed and a part-time student. Brent appeared to be a healthy child and was appropriately apprehensive during examination, which was unremarkable. Urinalysis was normal.

Because of the length of symptoms and the obvious concern of Mrs. Clark, the clinician thought further tracking questions were appropriate. Questions designed to track symptoms (see Chapter 3) and address the family developmental issues were asked. What happens when Brent wets his bed? Who tends to him? Who cleans up? What happens next? What does his father think about the problem? Have you discussed this together? What happens when you discuss it? How is discipline managed with Brent? What happens if he disobeys you? How does he respond to Mr. Clark's methods? How does he respond to your methods? How have Brent's symptoms affected the family? How much time do you have for yourself? How much time together do you have with your husband?

Mrs. Clark's answers suggested that Brent was triangulated in the center of a seemingly unconscious parental battle over who was the better parent. Brent's father (by Mrs. Clark's observation) arrived home from work and spent a little time with "his little girl" (Brent's sister). Eventually he asked Mrs. Clark if she had talked to Brent about the bedwetting. Mr. and Mrs. Clark gradually began to argue over how to stop the bedwetting with Mr. Clark advocating "spanking Brent for his stubbornness," and Mrs. Clark feeling she must protect Brent. By not saying or doing anything about the bedwetting, she thought she avoided upsetting Brent. Mrs. Clark expressed a lot of frustration about having to clean up the bed and protect Brent, as well as with Mr. Clark's attitude about the whole problem. She said her own patience was wearing thin and she was now unable to get Brent to obey in other routine matters. Her discipline techniques were those of repeated requests until angry, then a verbal outburst, and then completing the requested task herself. Mr. Clark's seemed to be uninvolved until he saw what he thought was stubbornness or disobedience, then he spanked Brent angrily.

On the basis of this information it seemed reasonable that a number of issues were complicating the bedwetting scenario. First of all, Mr. and Mrs. Clark needed some information on the prevalence and natural history of enuresis. Mrs. Clark was feeling like a failure as a mother because of Brent's bedwetting and was concerned that this might mean Brent had a serious emotional problem. Mr. and Mrs. Clark were not working together to address the issues. In fact, the bedwetting item had become the focus of a continued power struggle. Mrs. Clark was overly involved in Brent's life, which served as a strong source of mutual nurture and frustration. Mr. Clark seemed only peripherally involved with Mrs. Clark or Brent. His family time was spent with the daughter. There seemed to be little couple or fun time. In spite of this, Brent appeared to be a fairly happy and healthy child, implying the resources were present to manage this issue successfully if they could be tapped effectively.

This case could have been handled in several ways that might actually worsen the dysfunctional family dynamic. The physician might have replied after initial exam and history, "There's nothing physically wrong with Brent." From Mrs. Clark's viewpoint the physician could be perceived as saying that (a) Brent is emotionally disturbed (b) she and Mr. Clark are being manipulated, or (c) she is inadequate as a mother. Any of these interpretations might inflame an already tense overinvolvement with Brent's symptoms and possibly lead to more counterproductive "convincing" behaviors (the doctor trying to prove "Brent's just trying to get attention," Mrs. Clark trying to prove the doctor wrong, Brent developing more impressive symptoms, etc.).

Another drawback of saying that nothing is physically wrong with Brent might be the clinician's falsely reassuring himself and the family. In the first place it could be inaccurate, because the child may very well prove to have additional problems to his symptoms that are inapparent at the moment. More importantly, something is most definitely wrong from the point of view of the patient and his family or they would not consult a physician.

While the symptoms may seem to be a child just "trying to get attention," the most relevant question is "Why does this child seek more attention?" If simply told there is nothing wrong, Mrs. Clark may decide the physician is mistaken. She may then seek a different specialist's opinion, pushing for more and more testing until something shows up, perhaps an irrelevant finding like a "small bladder."

In Brent's case, Mrs. Clark was told, "I understand that Brent wets the bed and that you are concerned about this. From my findings I am reasonably certain Brent does not have anything medically serious. I want to do a few tests, which I expect to be normal, but I want you and Mr. Clark to come in so that we can have his opinion about Brent's symptoms, and that we can together decide the way to manage this." At this point if the bedwetting persists, then Brent and his family may be referred, or the physician may work with a family-oriented consultant, or he/she may see the family alone. By utilizing this approach, the physician avoids inflaming an already tense situation and raises the possibility of successfully addressing related life cycle issues (35,36).

Stage IV—Families with School-age Children (Ages 6–12)

The family with school-age children must negotiate the tasks of modifying boundaries to accommodate the growth (emotional and physical) of family members, and the assumption of new responsibilities by growing family members.

By going to school, children experience other adults, other rules, other patterns of behavior, and other children. This involves exploring new areas and challenging old boundaries. ("But Kim's mom said it was okay.") As a result of this input, the family system (rules, patterns, beliefs) are challenged and may change (8,21,22,24).

Along with redefined boundaries, different expectations are typically placed upon children and parents. Children are expected to take over more self-care (hygiene, dressing, feeding). Parents usually allow and encourage this assumption of responsibility. Some families expect members to accept responsibility for chores such as housework and for helping with other children. The family system is also changing, and the couple bond is now developing more elaborate executive functions (administration, task assignments, transportation, discipline, etc.). The clinical relevance of typical boundary and responsibility issues is illustrated by the next example.

Clinical Example #4: Shifting Boundaries

Joy is a 12-year-old who presented with the chief complaint of abdominal pain over the past 3 months. She described the pain as a "gnawing and aching" in the "pit of my stomach" that occurs day and night and is relieved by food. Joy noted some nausea, but no other symptoms. She was previously told by a doctor that she "may have an ulcer" and was placed on Maalox, which seemed to help for a few weeks. She was in good health otherwise and review of systems was negative. Joy was the oldest of three children, with a 10-year-old sister and an 8-year-old brother. Her parents were in good health. The mother worked full-time as a nurse, and father was a self-employed businessman. Joy's grades in school this year were not as good as previously. Her school attendance was good. On the abdominal exam epigastric tenderness was noted, but no guarding or rebound tenderness. Stool was positive for occult blood. An upper gastrointestinal tract series revealed a small duodenal ulcer.

Questions were asked of Joy's parents to explore the potential connection between life cycle issues and symptoms. Who sets the limits (bed time, homework, having friends over)? How are they set? Are they ever changed? How? What responsibilities does Joy have around the home? What are consequences if she carries them out? If she doesn't? What has happened since Joy has been sick? At school? At home? How has it affected the family? How has it affected your relationship as spouses and your roles of parents?

In this case Joy had adopted a parental role in this family—taking care of the younger children and functioning on the same authority or power level with her father. Joy and her mother constantly argued (like sisters); her father would occasionally respond with a "laying down of the law" that lasted 1 or 2 days. Since Joy had been sick the mother and father had further retreated from their executive parent role and avoided any conflict with Joy because the previous doctor said not to upset her.

Understanding that conflict over boundary issues was predictable in this family, the physician subsequently questioned the family and identified a dynamic of conflict avoidance ("We're a close family"). Such closeness generated a stressful environment of conflict avoidance that influenced

the development of an ulcer in Joy (29,32). In addition to the usual medicine, management was directed toward reestablishing the parental subsystem (mother and father getting together) and working out satisfactory
expectations for Joy (school, home, curfew). During the process of working
together with respect to Joy's symptoms, they were incidentally developing
their own communication, support, and bond (8,21,23). The counseling
portion of this management was done in conjunction with a family therapist. Working with a family therapist can be a productive arrangement
for the primary care physician who learns to recognize when the family
system is playing a significant role in the illness. Such an arrangement
also may enhance one's ability to recognize when to refer or ask for consultation in such cases (35,36).

Stage V—Families with Teenagers

Redefining boundaries further, assuming more new responsibilities by
growing youth, and the family's preparing for the departure of the offspring
are the tasks that face families with teenagers. The process of boundary
challenge begun in Stage IV now intensifies greatly as teenagers explore
many things and challenge family boundaries. As they mature, more expectations are placed upon the adolescents and more responsibility grant-
ed. This is an "up and down," "forward and backward" process of learning for both children and parents ("How much can they handle? How
much should they handle?") (2,8,21,24). During this period the family
anticipates the launch of the young adult out of the home and into the
world. Preparation includes encouraging self-reliance in the children, and
investing time in activities other than parenting, such as individual hobbies,
work, or activities as a couple (2,8,33,34). All of this occurs in most families
with considerable chaos and friction, with frequent mistakes, and with
numerous crises, as illustrated below.

Clinical Example #5: Impending Launch

Susan, a 16-year-old, was brought in by her mother, Mrs. Anderson, to the family
physician's office. Mrs. Anderson requested to see the physician alone while Susan
waited in the examining room. Mrs. Anderson very anxiously stated that she was
concerned that Susan was hanging around with "the wrong crowd." She was also
concerned that Susan was drinking too much alcohol. She stated she "didn't know
what had gotten into Susan, she used to be so nice and now we fight constantly."
She requested that the physician "talk to Susan, and straighten her out." The
physician went in to see Susan, who was sitting quietly in the examining room.
There was no particular evidence of substance abuse, although Susan was not
very talkative.

Susan refused to discuss any of these questions and chose to sit in silence. The physician offered to see Mrs. Anderson and Susan at a later
time when she and the physician had more time. While Mrs. Anderson

agreed readily, Susan still did not reply; however, both returned. Mr. Anderson, in a telephone conversation with the physician, refused to come. Questions prompted by family life cycle issues were asked. Who sets limits at home? How are they determined? Do they change? What responsibilities does Susan have at home? How are they determined? What's going to happen when Susan leaves home in a few years? Where is Susan's father? What does he say about what's going on? From observing the interaction between Susan and her mother and noting Mrs. Anderson's responses to the above questions, it was evident that (a) Mrs. Anderson was overinvolved in Susan's life, (b) Mr. Anderson was disengaged (seldom mentioned or involved), and (c) Mrs. Anderson was not prepared for Susan's impending departure from home. Upon direct questioning she expressed some anxiety about it. It was unclear how much of an issue substance abuse actually was, but this could be further explored in terms of the family system issues.

Management was aimed at supporting Mrs. Anderson's defining explicit and reasonable limits and placing expectations on Susan (allowance, homework, curfew, housework). In order for Susan to rebel, to express her differentness and dissatisfaction in some areas, Mrs. Anderson needed support as a functional single parent (since her husband was uninvolved). Susan was offered an active role in negotiating the limits, with the understanding that if she refused to participate, Mrs. Anderson would set limits that she thought best. Susan's mother was also encouraged to recognize her own limits ("Can you, Mrs. Anderson, police a 16-year-old 24 hours a day?"). In individual visits with Mrs. Anderson the physician encouraged discussion of plans and changes once Susan left home (2,8,9,21,24,33,34).

It is important that the clinician did not lecture Susan about her behavior. Lectures are rarely, if ever, effective over an extended period of time with any patient. In a situation like this, a clinician may tend to automatically side with either the parental authority figure or the adolescent seeking independence, undermining his/her effectiveness with both in the long run. The clinician in this case did not side with either Mrs. Anderson or Susan, but explored the problems using the family life cycle and then acted as facilitator for both to resolve essential issues.

Stage VI—Family Dispersion

Stage VI is characterized by the departure of the children from the family nest. It begins with the leaving of the first child and continues through the exit of the last. Many families get stuck to some extent in this stage, having one or more children who have difficulty leaving due to the emotional stuck-togetherness of the family members (22,23). The developmental tasks involve (a) the departure of the children and the attendant issues that enable it to occur, and (b) renegotiating the couple bond. When people enter and leave families, changes occur and adjustments are required, even if the whole event is viewed positively. When children leave home, the couple bond changes (2,8,21,24,33,34). Both parents may spend less time in a parent role, and thus have more time to invest in other ways, either together or separately. There are no prescriptive rules that define how two people negotiate such a transition successfully. Some require a lot of talking and planning, others seem to quietly adapt. Some couples get more involved with each other, some less involved. In any event, the departure of children changes the family and the couple responds.

Predictable crises may occur when the children do not leave home (at the appropriate age) or even when they do (the empty nest syndrome) (33,34). When a child returns home (or never leaves), leaving may become more difficult. If the child continues to stay beyond the cultural or societal norm, then there must be support in the system for the child's staying; i.e., either the mother or father or both are supporting the child's "no launch" position (21–24). They may do this unconsciously and in the role of "just being a good parent", i.e., doing the laundry, buying clothes and food, providing shelter, meals, and so forth. Conflict arises when one member of this triangle disagrees covertly or openly with the system continuing indefinitely and wants a change, while other members want to maintain the status quo. Perhaps even more importantly, the unlaunched member cannot individuate adequately while still glued to the family of origin (21–24).

Research suggests the empty nest syndrome may be the exception rather than the rule, although those exceptions may be the ones who present clinically. In fact, the attitude that most frequently accompanies this transition appears to be more of a positive sense of relief and freedom than that of a negative sense of loss (33,34). The clinician can learn to recognize those families who are high risk for experiencing difficulty in making the transition, i.e., those with an unsatisfying marital relationship and overattachment to one or more children, as in the following example.

Clinical Example #6: Leaving Home

Mrs. Davis, a 50-year-old woman, presented with a chief complaint of nervousness and sleep disturbance. She said she had been a nervous person all her adult life, but during the past 2 or 3 months she had noted an increase in symptoms, especially with sleep disturbance. She was often unable to go to sleep. Most nights, she awakened very early, unable to return to sleep. She described feeling sad but had no idea why she felt so sad and anxious. She had no weight loss or appetite loss. Mrs. Davis had been married for 30 years. She had one child 17 years of age, a senior at a local high school, who was to graduate and leave for college in 6 months. She described her husband as "a hard-working, quiet man who keeps to himself." Mrs. Davis had a generally healthy appearance. She seemed to be moderately anxious, with tense facial muscles, nervous smile, and a strained look constantly on her face. The remainder of the physical exam was normal.

Mrs. Davis was asked about family life cycle issues and systemic questions (see Chapter 3). What happens when you cannot sleep? How does it affect other family members? How does it affect your spouse? Your sex life? What is going to happen if these symptoms do not stop? What are your thoughts about your daughter's going off to college? How do you feel about it? What will change as a result of her leaving?

In responding to these questions, Mrs. Davis confirmed the physician's hunch that she was preoccupied with her daughter's leaving, but she was unaware of this being related to her difficulty sleeping. She expressed sadness over her daughter's leaving, which she had not discussed with either her daughter or her spouse. She expressed disgust with herself for not handling this "on my own," which was a pattern for her (harsh self-criticism).

The physician recommended the temporary use of a mild sedative to aid sleep, and requested a visit with the whole family. After seeing the Davis family together once, Mr. and Mrs. Davis came for several visits by themselves. The stated agenda at these sessions was (a) to discuss how things would change once their daughter is gone, and (b) to involve the husband and wife in solving the wife's sleep disturbance problem. The husband suggested that she awaken him when she could not sleep and talk with him. This helped decrease her anxiety and the frequency of sleep disturbance. Once this family addressed these issues, Mrs. Davis' sleep disturbance improved, although she occasionally still had a restless night. She found the temporary use of a sleep aid helpful and became able to manage without them after a few months. The couple planned more couple activities and eventually made the transition over a 1-year period.

Mrs. Davis' sleep disturbance and anxiety were connected to her perception of her daughter's leaving and her anticipatory grief about that event. Her anxiety was further increased by her feeling unable to discuss this with either her daughter or her husband, who seemed to her to be unconcerned. When asked during a family interview how they felt about the daughter's impending move from home, the daughter and Mr. Davis expressed some anxiety similar to Mrs. Davis'. This normalized Mrs. Davis' symptoms somewhat and she began to see herself as going through a normal transition, rather than being sick or weak (8,21,24).

One goal of management was to help Mrs. Davis find a way to control symptoms (insomnia, nervousness, etc.). The physician did not tell her that "Everything is going to be just fine, you'll see," or that she would never be anxious again. Absolute cure of these types of symptoms is unlikely and such a promise sets the stage for another disappointment. Improvement in symptoms, however, is a less ambitious objective and raises the probability of success. The physician told Mrs. Davis, "These kinds of symptoms affect your function in the family. I would like to talk with you and other members of the family and hear their opinions regarding these symptoms. I am recommending some laboratory tests that I think will be normal. In the long run, I think that together we can find a way for you to manage with these symptoms."

There is sometimes a knee-jerk inclination to treat all anxiousness with anxiolytic agents without really probing for the reasons a person is anxious. In this case, while Mrs. Davis described herself as a basically nervous person, she had a recent increase in symptoms. Treating her symptoms pharmacologically without also exploring the causes and offering thera-peutic counseling would be like giving an analgesic for chest pain without considering and treating the cause of the pain. Anxiolytics may complicate recognition or proper management of depression. Tranquilizers also may dim the anxiousness that is sometimes needed as a motivating force for change. In other words, if Mrs. Davis experiences no anxiety, how mo-tivated will she be to work at making the transition presented by her daughter's leaving home? The temporary administration of mild sedative in this case enabled Mrs. Davis to get some rest, regain some sense of control, and become a better problem solver.

Stage VII—The Older Couple

The developmental tasks for the last stage of the family life cycle are (a) facing retirement, (b) facing each other, and (c) facing the issues of aging and death.

Couples may either look forward to or dread retirement, but generally the system changes in some way (work expectations or schedule, fixed income, slowing down, etc.). Without children, the couple has more time that was formerly spent in the parent role. Two people may feel thrown together who had only seen each other in passing for several years. Some-times women are still employed and the male spouse has retired, which presents a different system than previously (and maybe role reversal). The couple must face the tasks of aging. Caring for elderly parents, dealing with physical limitations and more frequent illnesses or hospitalizations become part of the daily tasks of life (2,7,8,11,13,24).

Clinical Example #7: Retirement Pains

Mrs. Johnson, a 60-year-old woman, presented with back pain. She had a long history of chronic back pain with previous work-up including X-rays and physical examination that revealed a lordotic curvature susceptible to strain. She was somewhat overweight and, with aging, her back pain had intermittently flared up. It had been more persistent now for several months, although no more intense, and she had no new symptoms. While she talked about her back pain, she looked somewhat sad and frustrated. Upon questioning, Mrs. Johnson described feeling generally worse since Mr. Johnson's retirement.

She stated that he is always "under foot." He had organized her kitchen and was taking over the house. She described him as having found new energy in his retirement and enjoying the application of his business skills at home. She found notes on the cabinets and refrigerator regarding rules to make the home run smoothly. However, Mrs. Johnson, despite the fact she had more free time now, was feeling generally worse and specifically guilty about not appreciating this help. She noted more concern about her adult daughters and their marriages and children.

In fact, she found herself constantly calling, visiting, or worrying about her daughters and their families. She was becoming more and more depressed as Mr. Johnson was doing more and more at home.

This family illustrates several issues that often occur in clinical practice. Mrs. Johnson's symptoms were connected to changes in her family system. Due to Mr. Johnson's retirement and his adaptation, she was now unemployed as both mother and housewife. Second, Mr. Johnson's adjustment, if viewed independently, appeared healthy. If viewed from the systems approach, however, the family has a problem. Another notable event followed Mrs. Johnson's increase in anxiety, that is, her return to a role (mothering) both familiar and comfortable to her. At this stage of the family life cycle, however, mothering was inappropriate and created more problems for her daughters and their families than it solved.

Several potentially useful management options are available. If indicated by history and physical exam (major criteria for depression, weight loss, etc.), antidepressant medication may be helpful. In addition, Mr. and Mrs. Johnson might both come to discuss changes and expectations and responsibilities since retirement. Further counseling may be conducted by a physician with such training or through referral to, or in consultation with, a family therapist.

Limitations and Hazards

There are some limitations and potential drawbacks to utilizing the family life cycle concept in practice. As one might expect, families may be in more than one stage at a time. A couple who recently married, for instance, each having children from a previous marriage, and who have a newborn are in family formation (Stage I), childbearing (Stage II), and school-age children (Stage IV) stages simultaneously.

The second problem is that the issues in some patient encounters may not fit well in the life cycle framework. The family life cycle is a helpful way to organize and view events and perhaps sort out the issues. The only real difference the concept makes is in the clinician's and family's understanding of the problem. Therefore, one cannot force a patient into the concept ("I *know* you *must* be upset about your son's going off to college.") The patient's reason for consulting a physician may have little to do with the family life cycle.

Another hazard is the temptation in medicine to look only for one all-encompassing, straightforward cause of symptoms. In fact, symptoms are almost always the product of numerous factors, and the biopsychosocial model addresses them as such (27,29). Therefore, the orientation suggested here is not simplistic ("Aha! Your headaches are due to your husband's retirement.") Rather a contextual and multifactorial view of symptoms is suggested, i.e., more than one factor can be contributing to the illness. Consideration of the family life cycle may help address some of those factors. This model does not diminish the importance of the history and physical examination, a thorough neurological examination, and appropriate laboratory tests. On the other hand, neither is it best used only after all other work-up is negative. It is most useful when integrated with other clinical assessment tools in an effort to arrive at the most complete, accurate diagnosis and best management.

Finally, besides the normal and predictable crises encountered in the family life cycle, people also experience unpredictable crises—disability, premature death, accidents, illness, and divorce, among others. These kinds of events have been correlated with the risk of significant illness. Information about life events cannot be neatly quantified with individual patients ("Forty-one percent of your ulcer is due to your divorce."), but it is nonetheless important to accurate assessment and effective management. At times, unpredictable crises can make it particularly difficult for families to cope when they coincide with vulnerable times in the family life cycle or with toxic issues in a given family. While using the family life cycle to address predictable crises, one needs to consider the influence of unpredictable events and toxic family issues as well.

Summary

The family life cycle is a series of stages of family development, with developmental tasks and crises characteristic of each stage. There are advantages, limitations, and precautions for using this concept in medical practice. The family life cycle can be a useful instrument to help the physician understand (a) the predictable family issues, (b) the distress that can accompany these issues, and (c) the possibility of a relationship between these issues and the patient's chief complaint. Utilizing the life cycle approach leads to a more accurate depiction of illnesses and families. Its use enhances the practice of medicine by recognizing and incorporating a human dimension that otherwise may be overlooked.

References

1. Loomis CP, Hamilton CH: Family life cycle analysis. Social Forces, 1936;15(December):225–231.
2. Duvall EM: Marriage and Family Development, ed 5. Philadelphia, Lippincott, 1977.
3. Hill R: Families under Stress. Westport, CT, Greenwood Press, 1979.
4. Glick PC: The family cycle. Am J Sociol 1947;12:164–174.
5. Glick PC: Updating the life cycle of the family. J Marriage Fam 1977;39(2):5–13.
6. Feldman H, Feldman M: The family life cycle: Some suggestions for recycling. J Marriage Fam 1975;37(5):277–284.
7. Gould R: The phases of adult life: A study in developmental psychology. Am J Psychiatry 1972;129(5):33–34.

8. Carter E, McGoldrick M: The Family Life Cycle. New York, Gardner Press, 1980.
9. Solomon M: A developmental, conceptual premise for family therapy. Fam Process 1973;12:179–188.
10. Erikson E: Childhood and Society, ed 2. New York, Norton, 1963, pp 247–274.
11. Neugarten BL: Adult personality: Toward a psychology of the life cycle, in Neugarten BL (ed) *Middle Age and Aging*. Chicago, The University of Chicago Press, 1968.
12. Levinson DJ, Darrow CN, Klein EB, et al: The Seasons of A Man's Life. New York, Knopf, 1978, pp 18–39.
13. Levinson DJ: The mid-life transition: A period in adult psychosocial development. Psychiatry 1977;40:99–102.
14. Sheehy G: Passages. New York, Dutton, 1976.
15. Medalie JH: Family Medicine Principles and Application. Baltimore, Williams & Wilkins, 1978, pp 111–212.
16. Rakel RE: Principles of Family Medicine. Philadelphia, Saunders, 1977, pp 279–304.
17. Medalie JH: The family life cycle and its implication for family practice. J Fam Pract 1979;9:47–56.
18. Johnson HC: Working with stepfamilies: Principles of practice. Social Work, July, 1980. Vol. 25, No. 4 pp. 304–308.
19. Talbot Y: The reconstituted family. Can Fam Physician 1981;27:103–1807.
20. Minuchin S, Montalvo B, Guerney BG Jr, Rosman BL, Schumer F: Families of the Slums. New York, Basic Books, 1967.
21. Minuchin S: Families and Family Therapy. Cambridge, MA, Harvard University Press, 1974.
22. Bowen M: The use of family theory in clinical practice. Comprehens Psychiatry 1966;17:345–374.
23. Bowen M: Family Therapy in Clinical Practice. New York, Jason Aronson, 1978.
24. Satir V: Conjoint Family Therapy. Palo Alto, CA, Science and Behavior Books, 1964.
25. Brody H: The systems view of man: Implications for medicine, science, and ethics. Perspect Biol Med 1973 17(Autumn):71–92.
26. Engel GL: The clinical application of the biopsychosocial model. Am J Psychiatry 1980;137:535–544.
27. Engel GL: The need for a new medical model: A challenge for biomedicine. Science 1977;196;129–136.
28. Schmidt D: Family determinants of disease: Depressed lymphocyte function following the loss of a spouse. Fam Sys Med 1983;1(1):33–39.
29. Ackerman SH, et al: Recent separation and the onset of peptic ulcer disease in older children and adolescents. Psychosom Med 1981;43:305–310.
30. Holmes TH, Rahe RH: The social readjustment scale. J Psychosom Res 1967;11:213–218.
31. Minuchin S, Baker L, Rosman B, Liebman R, Milman L, Todd TC: A conceptual model of psychosomatic illness in children. Arch Gen Psychiatry 1975;32:1031–1038.
32. Doherty WJ, Baird MA: Family Therapy and Family Medicine. New York, Guilford Press, 1983.

33. Harkins EB: Effects of empty nest transition on self report of psychological and physical well-being. J Marriage Fam 1978;40:549–556.
34. Lowenthal MF, Chiriboga D: Transition to the empty nest—crisis, challenge, or relief. Arch Gen Psychiatry 1972;26:8–14.
35. Crouch MA, Davis TC: Working with families: I. Basic family oriented health care, in *Textbook of Family Medicine*. Chicago, Yearbook Medical Publishers.
36. Glenn ML, Atkins L, Singer R: Integrating a family therapist into a family medical practice. Fam Syst Med 1984;2(2), pp. 137–145.

CHAPTER 5

Families and Illness

Lisa Baker

The vast majority of patients have families who share in the decision making and consequences of an illness. In fact, the involvement of family members when someone is ill is so common that their absence should raise some concerns. This chapter first describes the decision-making processes that occur involving the patient, the family, and the health care team. Second, the chapter traces the family's experience of an illness from its onset to its conclusion in recovery or death, and suggestions are made for therapeutic interventions by health care providers.

Clinical Decision Making

The Health Care Team

Clinical decision making as a process begins when clinician and patient meet. First, the duration and severity of the presenting problem are evaluated by history taking and physical examination. As information is gathered, factors are weighed, hypotheses are formulated, and plans are developed for diagnosis, treatment, and patient education. Besides the current symptoms, the patient's past medical history is considered, especially any previous treatment of the symptoms. The combining of these facts into a good decision is usually relatively informal, though in some cases it can be a formal, precise process that relies on mathematical formulas that weight various factors based on research. In appendicitis, for example, the five factors that are important in the decision to remove an appendix are each assigned a precise number (1). Combining the numbers for all the factors supports either a decision to operate or a decision to continue to observe the patient for the time being. Other contextual factors, such as time and available resources, also enter into clinical decision making. (If one waits, how likely is it that the patient's condition will worsen? Is a consultant readily available? Is a hospital bed available? Can the patient afford the necessary treatment? Is the patient willing to be admitted to the hospital now?) Making these decisions effectively is the crux of the clinician's role.

The Patient and the Family

Just as clinicians make decisions about diagnosis and management, patients and families have their own decision-making processes. Their processes begin much earlier than the clinician's and continue after the patient and family leave the health care system. Families' encounters with health care professionals are only interludes, albeit sometimes critical ones, in their complicated lives. While patients also evaluate symptoms in light of their medical history, time factors, and available resources, there is one important difference, i.e., the *context* in which they evaluate symptoms. This difference may cause them to weight factors quite differently than the clinician would.

Patients and their families have gone through at least three steps before they encounter clinicians: (a) symptoms have occurred and have become a problem; (b) someone has defined the patient as sick enough to need help beyond the care that can be given at home; and (c) someone has chosen a time and place of entry into the health care system (emergency room, clinic, phone call, etc.). As consumers of health care, families must deal with such practicalities as cost, transportation, medical records, and insurance—things that can be significant barriers. Prior experience with clinic personnel, hospital staffs, billing offices, and insurance companies tempers their decisions. A bad experience in an emergency room may mean that they will call a physician at home next time. A series of positive encounters with a clinic staff and a physician may ensure that they will make extra efforts to come for scheduled clinic appointments, or regularly attend prenatal classes.

People's roles in the family and at work also influence how they make decisions about seeking health care. In more traditional families, mothers are indispensable and rarely get sick. Even if they feel sick, they assume the sick role with great reluctance and tend not to interrupt their tasks to seek medical care. Men, on the other hand, seek health care less than women do, partly because of the financial need to work and partly because of the association of "sickness" with "weakness." As more families include single adults or both spouses as earners, some changes in health care decision-making patterns may be expected. These families are often stretched taut and can barely manage when someone gets sick. If support from extended family members, friends, or neighbors is unavailable in times of crisis, such families can decompensate.

Disagreement or Agreement about Patient Care

Families vary in the judgments that they make in caring for a family member, and health care professionals may get frustrated when a patient's judgments are different from their own. For example, a physician may be annoyed when a patient calls in the middle of the night about a baby who is sick for the first time. The parents may be labeled as overanxious or overprotective because their criteria for the decision to make the call are different than those of the doctor. On the other end of the spectrum, when a woman fails to come in for her yearly Pap smear, she may be thought of as negligent and irresponsible. Although this might be the case, her decision not to come in may be based on other factors not taken into account in the physician's decision-making model. In a recent case, a 25-year-old black woman quit coming in for pelvic exams and Pap smears after a consistent record of yearly checkups. When she finally came in after two and a half years, the nurse learned that her mother had died suddenly of cancer, and the woman was frightened that she might be found to have the disease. Even though she had no symptoms, it took a number of months for the woman to be willing to take the risk of being evaluated for cancer.

Families and clinicians may agree or disagree in their decision-making about patient care, and these feelings can be expressed in overt or covert ways. Figure 5.1 gives some examples of how families may express themselves. Families who disagree with the clinician's plan may doctor-shop, leave the hospital against medical advice, bring a lawsuit, or openly disagree and try to negotiate. Covert ways of expressing differences would be noncompliance, attempts at manipulation, or criticizing the professional to other people without his/her knowledge. When families and the health care team agree on the patient's care, families may compliment clinicians and recommend them to other people. More passive or covert ways of expressing consensus are to be compliant, to return for future health care, and to have no complaints.

When they feel uncomfortable with decisions made by others, families may tend to respond in less confrontive ways because they feel relatively powerless. Because many patients and families see themselves as having

	Disagreement about Patient Care	Agreement about Patient Care
Overt Expression	Leave hospital against medical advice (AMA) "Doctor-shop" Negotiate or complain Sue	Referrals Compliments
Covert Expression	Noncompliance Criticism to outsiders Manipulation	Compliance No complaints Returning for future health care

FIGURE 5.1.   Styles of family expression in clinical decision making with the health care team.

few choices and little power, and therefore minimal responsibility for participating in their health care, it is important for the clinician to recognize conflict as a signal to check out possible disagreement about patient care. Assumptions may need to be clarified and goals renegotiated. For example, one family agreed that a certain family member needed to have invasive tests to see if she had metastatic lung cancer. When diagnosis was positively established, however, they disagreed with the doctors about using aggressive chemotherapy, preferring to maintain quality of life at the price of some possible loss of quantity of life. They passively resisted the physicians' plan by not bringing the patient in for her treatments, an action that the doctors misinterpreted as negligence and lack of understanding. This situation might have been avoided if there had been a conference with the patient, the family, and the health care team in which these feelings were aired and the decision was openly negotiated. A routine approach of meeting with the family may prevent crises over "no code" orders, intubations, or prolonged, expensive hospital stays.

Family Systems and the Illness Process

In exploring the experiences of families with an ill member, family processes, family strengths, and possible therapeutic interventions for each phase of illness will be examined. This discussion will follow the stages of acute phase, treatment onset, chronic phase, and recovery or deterioration (see Table 5.1). The description is not intended to be exhaustive, but merely illustrative of some common interaction patterns of families and health care professionals.

Acute Phase

When illness onset is acute, as in the case of a sudden heart attack, the family may shift into roles and tasks for handling a crisis that, in some cases, are aimed at helping the person survive. During this time, the family tends to close ranks and draw closer to each other. They generally perceive the illness as something outside that is threatening the patient and/or the family. Stress theory is often used to conceptualize this acute phase. Not only do patients face an event or events that are stressful, but families also face stress stemming from the onset of an illness in the family.

One model of family stress and adaptation that has been applied to illness is the "Family Adaptation Adjustment Response" or FAAR model (2). This model builds on the initial work of Hill (3), who developed the ABCX model to describe individuals' reactions to stress: A (stressor event) interacts with B (the family's resources), which interacts with C (the definition of the event by the family), which produces X (the crisis). The FAAR model expands on these basic factors and highlights stressful family events, definitions, resources, and coping styles. Based on these factors, family coping would also be influenced by other stresses accompanying

TABLE 5.1. Family systems and the illness process.

Illness sequence	Family processes	Family strengths	Therapeutic interventions
Acute phase	Crisis management—survival Family closes ranks Stress balanced against resources Purging effect	Strong emotional and practical resources Absence of other life changes or stressful events	Crisis intervention Assess family patterns Provide comfort Networking Provide information
Treatment onset	Family becomes disabled Adherence to medical regimen Vulnerable to coalitions with doctors and staff Negative feelings toward medical staff	Economic adequacy Family cooperation Problem-solving skills Clear generational boundaries and coalitions Shared leadership Clear self-responsible communication	Avoid triangulation with families Establish clear boundaries Frank, direct information for all family members, including children
Chronic phase	Illness becomes stable Reorganization of family Illness becomes regulator Development may be arrested Emotional adjustment out of sync	Strong parent coalition Clear, self-responsible communication Clear boundaries Humor, warmth, affection	Encourage strong parent coalition Clear, self-responsible communication Recognize isolation or misplaced conflict Refer if necessary Target unsuccessful behaviors
Recovery	Rigid roles become problematic Convergent/divergent styles Treatment for behavioral problems Illness changes—ambiguity, marginality Patient recovers, family may not	Flexibility of roles Negotiation skills Explicit expectations	Communicate clear expectations Predict typical setbacks Normalize negative feelings Differentiate between poor coping vs. coping well with difficult situation
Deterioration	"Unfinished business" "Secrets uneasily held" May minimize illness or may neglect other responsibilities	Flexibility of coping patterns Ability to release patient and mourn	Reframe passive denial Recognize scapegoating and "hidden patients" Normalize negative feelings Allow family to mourn

the illness. For example, a young man's impending death from a clotting deficiency causing hemorrhage was much more traumatic for his middle-age mother because it occurred 1 month after the death of her own mother and 6 months after her brother died. Another family, struggling to retain their home on the mother's salary after the father lost his job at an automobile factory, saw the grandfather's stroke as the final straw.

How the family explains or interprets the illness may have much to do with how they handle this acute phase. In one family a mother and grandmother brought a previously undiagnosed 14-year-old girl into the emergency room in very serious condition with ketoacidosis. The grandmother was hysterical, and the mother was panic stricken. However, later in an illness, this is seldom the case. After a family has had a number of experiences with ketoacidosis in a diabetic member, they may respond with appropriate concern, relative indifference, or anger instead of panic when an episode occurs. Thus, families' perceptions of the critical nature of an event may differ markedly during the course of the illness. Members of the health care team can help shape the family's definition of an event by the way they communicate their own perception of the illness. Some families need to increase their sense of urgency, and others need to be calmed. Health care professionals can give information and answer questions in a way that will alter the family's perception of the situation, for better or worse.

Some of the resources that a family brings to the stressful situation are tangible, including the practical things mentioned above, such as money, transportation, insurance, and good health care. Resources may also be intangible, such as helpful contacts in the bureaucracies with which families have to deal, job flexibility, confidence in their ability to handle things, and friendships. William Schroeder, the second artificial heart recipient, had Social Security, but it was his personal contact with President Reagan that made it possible for him to get through the red tape and promptly receive his money.

In the FAAR model, family strengths include strong emotional and practical resources and the absence of other stresses or life changes that might deplete the resources. One way for the health care team to intervene is to become an effective part of the family's resources. This may happen by channeling the family to appropriate community services and listening in a nondefensive way to family members expressing feelings that may identify the health care system as part of the problem instead of part of the solution.

A situation that is an acute medical crisis for the health care team is likely to be, in addition, an emotional crisis for the family and the patient. At these times the family's needs often may appear to be at odds with those of the medical personnel. The health care team needs to act quickly and efficiently at the very point when the family most needs information and emotional support. At other times this conflict of needs is less problematic. For example, the family's crisis may be at the time of diagnosis of an illness that is not immediately life-threatening, after a gradual coalescing of symptoms. When a 21-year-old patient and his family learn that he has multiple sclerosis, for example, the nurse and doctor can easily spend time with them, explaining the disease, answering questions, and listening to their anger and grief as it begins to be expressed.

Family behavior during an acute phase may be most fairly viewed as a snapshot of the family in unusual circumstances, not as a baseline of normal family functioning. The family may rise to the occasion and discover new bonds and ways of coping. The father may be taking primary responsibility for children for the first time, siblings may take care of each other, and people may have conversations about important things that usually go undiscussed. Alternatively, some families are stretched to the breaking point by serious illness. When Bob and Sue pledged at their wedding to be faithful "in sickness and in health," they never dreamed of adapting to a spinal cord injury that would result in quadriplegia, leaving Bob unable to work at the only job he knew how to do. Serious illness often has a purging effect on the family—it calls forth both the best and the worst.

Treatment Onset

As a treatment regimen begins, the family as well as the patient may become disabled. Treatment may require families to stay out of the way and be almost completely excluded at points, such as when the patient is in the intensive care unit. At other times, therapy may require families to be extraordinarily involved, as in home dialysis of renal patients. Paradoxically, in many cases of hospitalization, the more serious the patient's condition, the less time the patient and family have together during treatment. The message to family members that "there is nothing you can do, so you might as well go home and get some rest" may be well intentioned on the part of the clinician, but it may heighten the greatest despair felt by a family member, i.e., "there is nothing I can do."

It is easy for health care professionals to see the family as a nuisance—people to be placated or avoided if possible. They get in the way, they will not leave when they are supposed to, and they ask inappropriate questions. In reality, family members may be crucial to the treatment of a patient's illness. Studies have shown that designing treatment strategies that include the patient's family members improves patient outcome. This finding has been shown in conditions as diverse as cardiac-related high risk behaviors (4), adaptation to a hand-splint regimen for arthritis (5), schizophrenia (6), and dialysis during end-stage renal disease (7).

In this phase of assimilating medical regimens into their life-style—whether that means coming daily to visit the patient in the hospital or giving insulin shots at home—the family depends heavily on the medical staff for patient care and information. Especially when the patient is hospitalized, the family members may feel totally out of control of what is happening. Sometimes an action that seems to sabotage patient care may be an attempt by the patient or family member to regain some control. For example, the mother of a 13-year-old black boy exasperated the medical staff by refusing to let them get near her son after he was diagnosed as having leukemia. Families may turn their anger and frustration toward the staff, sometimes because they have legitimate contentions with the system, and other times because their anger at the disease is misdirected toward those caring for the patient. The other side of the coin is that family members can get overinvolved or overdependent on a staff person, and it is important to establish what are appropriate expectations. It may be flattering and rewarding to a physician to hear the family tell him/her that he/she is the only physician who can cure the patient. However, such comments may be an emotional setup when the patient is not cured and the physician has let them down.

The patient and the family are consumers of health care and information, and members of the health care team are powerful as providers of these things. In being an information broker, the clinician can easily become caught in the middle by communicating differently with different members of the family. For instance, to tell the family about the patient's health status and not to tell the patient is asking for trouble. This strategy only adds to the patient's feeling of being out of control. Likewise, family members may put the health care professional in the middle by telling him/her secrets or by using the person as a mediator. In one case, Kathy told her physician that her husband, Mark, had a drinking problem that was ruining their marriage, but requested that the physician pretend not to know. The physician responded to the disclosure with sympathy and promised not to bring it up. Kathy subsequently went home and used the physician's sympathetic response as "ammunition" against her husband, saying that the doctor was appalled and agreed that Mark should quit drinking.

A basic family strength that is important in the treatment phase is financial resources adequate to meet the needs. Without enough money, families are taxed beyond their ability to function well in other ways. Many families face the difficulty of allocating scarce resources between competing basic needs such as food, shelter, and utilities.

On an interpersonal level, family cooperation is crucial, including positive expectations for the patient and reinforcement of treatment progress. Maintaining clear boundaries both within and around the family is important, as is shared leadership between spouses. Direct family communication encourages good problem solving while patient care needs are being negotiated.

One facet of communication that is extremely important is the notion of self-responsibility. When people are sacrificing sleep, daily routines, recreation, and other necessities over a period of time, families can experience much strain. Families do better when their members talk to each other about what they want—not making demands, but telling each other their needs and desires and negotiating how everyone's needs can be met as well as can be managed. The health care team can model healthy communication by telling the family about their own thoughts, feelings, and limitations and by asking that the family do the same. An area in which communication is especially important is with children, who deserve frank and direct information as much as adults do.

Chronic Phase

As an illness wears on, families develop routines around hospital and office visits, altered diets, shifts in roles, and the like. In some cases, illness becomes stable and chronic, e.g., diabetes, chronic lung disease, or arthritis. Accordingly, many decisions, activities, and expectations center around the illness. Most families adapt heroically to illness, but occasionally their altered patterns may backfire. For some families, illness may become a regulator of family conflict. A wife may feel guilty and hesitate to express her anger at her husband, who is recovering from a heart attack. As a result, everyone habitually tiptoes around Dad and perhaps eventually explodes at him or at someone else in an inappropriate way. Minuchin et al. (8) described how this situation may develop among families with sick children. Billy has an asthma attack during a fight between his parents. The parents stop fighting and rush the child to the hospital. As this pattern repeats itself, the timing and duration of fights can become constrained by the asthma attacks and vice versa. If this pattern is not interrupted, several things may occur: (a) Mom and Dad never resolve their differences (cannot finish a fight); (b) Billy may get the idea that they must never fight or something bad will happen; (c) Billy may feel that he is the only one who can keep them from fighting and is responsible for doing so; (d) only when Billy is sick will Mom and Dad be reconciled; and (e) Billy's asthma will be poorly controlled: he will forget his medicine, emotional upset will trigger attacks, or one of his parents will forget his medicine. It will be difficult for the clinician to interact with Billy and his parents to control Billy's asthma in a straightforward way under such circumstances.

Minuchin et al. (8) referred to families where daily interaction becomes linked with illness episodes as psychosomatic families. In studies of anorexia nervosa, brittle diabetes, and asthma, some characteristic patterns of family behavior that emerge are: enmeshment, rigidity, overprotectiveness, and lack of conflict resolution. Members of these families are overly involved with one another (enmeshed), and the child tends to be triangulated between the mother and father. Patterns may develop with the child being overinvolved with one or both parents, or the child may be the regular target (scapegoat) for parental anger, allowing the parents to avoid dealing with their marital conflicts. The illness symptoms often command attention and preempt unresolved problems. Sometimes this painful equilibrium can go on for years, perpetuating both family discord and a child's illness.

During the chronic stage, the distinction between organic and psychosomatic illness becomes blurred. Every illness occurs in a social context; that is, the illness begins to have meaning and consequences in peoples' lives and feelings. In trying to adapt to changing circumstances, families may get stuck and maintain patterns that have outlived their usefulness. Secondary gain refers to getting something positive out of being ill or disabled. An illness can also bestow benefits upon family members as well as the patient. A person may get more attention, a break from home or work responsibilities, or a chance to reexamine life goals. Though these benefits may be constructive for all concerned, the term secondary gain usually carries a negative connotation. It implies that the ill person (or family member) is unnecessarily prolonging the sick role at others' expense because of what he/she gets out of it, regardless of how aware or unaware that person is of the role of secondary gain.

Another balancing act that the family must perform is to attend to the needs of the patient while trying to meet normal developmental needs of other family members. Problems may begin as the sick child gets more attention than siblings, or as the wife becomes the sole breadwinner for the family and the husband must face being dependent in unprecedented ways. Members of the health care profession may see this as the fallout from the continuous taxing demands of the illness.

On an emotional level, people may be "out of sync" with each other, some needing to avoid talking about the illness when others need to discuss it the most. The same process can happen within the health care team and in their interaction with the family. A nurse may be in a position to listen to the patient or family members voice some thoughts and feelings about the illness, but it may be at the very time when the nurse has reached his/her own limit of emotional expenditure. It is a delicate matter to negotiate the need to express or not express feelings, and most of that process happens implicitly through body language that says "I want to talk" or "I do not want to talk." While the patient usually moves faster than the family through various emotions of fear, sadness, and anger, family members also face those same feelings. The important thing is for people to experience these emotions with an appropriate intensity and timing and then move on. Because family members may be out of step with each other, one person may appear to be inappropriate to the rest and may be rebuffed by the family. In a family in which the teenage daughter, Dawn, was in a car wreck that left her in a coma for several weeks, the family was relieved and optimistic when she finally regained consciousness and began to talk again. Dawn, however, was overwhelmed with bitterness as her condition became clear to her. It took patience and understanding from the family to allow her the integrity of her own emotional process without demanding that she jump ahead to match their own.

Actually this rhythm of adaptation can be viewed as an asset in the family. When one person is unable to listen to the fear expressed by the patient or a family member about the future, another person can step in. One person's time of strength may be another's period of weakness or regrouping. Family members who recognize these differences in coping can draw on them as a strength instead of blaming each other for being insensitive when they do not respond in identical ways.

Guilt can play a big part in patients and families coming to grips with an illness. The nurse, doctor, or physician associate can encourage people to let go of regrets that seem unfounded and cause unnecessary distress. However, Tucker (9) has pointed out that, although health care professionals usually try to dispel guilt by rationally explaining causality of the disease, guilt can have a positive side to it. The fact that a person feels guilt implies that he/she feels some sense of mastery over life circumstances. This belief can be turned around to be an asset for mobilizing and motivating patients and families.

Families' grief can reflect multiple and simultaneous losses. Besides losing a degree of healthy functioning, the person may also lose previous roles that have meaning and practical benefit, such as breadwinner, athlete, or freelance businesswoman. Plans for the future may also be interrupted, for example, the intention to go back to work after a baby is born. A dual-career couple had a baby with spina bifida and had to deal with severe, sudden changes in their own career expectations and life-style along with their grief over the child's health and future.

The health care team can encourage family strengths during the chronic phase of an illness by relating to marriage partners as a team and by being alert for signs of scapegoating or misplaced conflict. Those who work closely in the situation can watch for isolation of some family members and the signs of family conflict. It is not the job of the health care team to "fix" the family, but, by being aware of problems, they can sometimes be more supportive and help the family fix itself. Many otherwise well-functioning families may develop problems when someone is ill, and these problems are usually temporary. A child may begin misbehaving at home or at school when a parent is in the hospital, but things usually return to normal when the illness ends. Health care professionals help these families by offering encouragement and reassurance that the situation is probably temporary, and by normalizing what is happening.

Just as a prior condition of diabetes can make an infection a much worse problem, when families who have a history of troubles are confronted with the additional stress of chronic illness, their problems often worsen. With these families, the medical team may intervene by offering counseling or referrals for in-depth therapy. Family conferences in the hospital are good places for discussion since it is easier to convene people at that time. Families may be more likely to seek and receive help during this period since the illness may push them beyond their limits of coping.

In attempting to adapt, families may persist in using unsuccessful methods of solving problems. In some cases the health care team can help the family interrupt these "vicious cycles." For example, a teenage boy, Patrick, was hospitalized and had no appetite. His mother got worried and frustrated after several days of his not eating. While she did everything she could think of to get him to eat, Patrick began to be annoyed and felt even less like eating. The issue became a power struggle between the two, not unlike other struggles they had had in a normal parent–teenager relationship. The nurse was able to relieve the mother of her responsibility to get the boy to eat and convinced her to use mealtimes as a chance to get some errands done. The nurse began to joke with Patrick and to make his eating a matter of his own control. After one more skipped meal, the boy began eating.

Recovery Phase

In time, some patients begin to recover from their illness, while others deteriorate. For patients that recover, there may be some difficulty in returning to normal roles. Just as there are costs and benefits for the patient and family in having someone in the sick role, there are also costs to returning to work and to family responsibilities. The family has had to reorganize to get along with limited or no help from the sick person, and now they have to adjust their patterns again as the person reenters the system.

It is in this stage, when the family believes that the patient's health is improving, that rigid roles and coalitions between family members may agitate to the point that the family seeks help for some problem, though it is seldom identified as illness related. In this sense, the patient recovers, but the family may not recover. Penn (10) discussed these families as systems that try to maintain old patterns and simultaneously try to develop new ones. She hears these families saying "We are behaving as if we are ongoing, but we may not be ongoing."

When Carol went to work for the first time after her husband, Jim, had a heart attack, she began to find some unexpected benefits in getting a paycheck, making new friends, and developing some skills. Although she wanted her husband to feel better, Carol found that she also wanted to continue her new life-style. However, there was conflict when she talked it over with Jim, since their marriage had been built around her being totally dependent on him. It had been hard for him to accept her working outside the home even temporarily, but for her to work permanently was quite threatening. The conflict would have been a difficult one to deal with even when both people were at their best. When Jim was still not feeling very well and Carol was weary from caring for him, the problems were exacerbated. Families have to develop considerable flexibility of roles and negotiation skills to be able to work through this kind of change.

Families have different styles of handling recovery. In Speedling's (11) study of heart attack victims, he noted two types of family role styles. In *convergent* families the patient is primary and roles are fairly rigid. This style tends to discourage the patient from early withdrawal from the sick role. For instance, a patient may be encouraged to stay in the hospital or at home longer than the physicians think is medically necessary, but the patient may benefit from more rigid roles that assure that his/her needs are attended to. *Divergent* families put more emphasis on individual needs of family members, which leads to earlier withdrawal from the sick role as well as more rapid recovery of normal roles for other family members.

The vulnerabilities of this style are that families tend to play down the limitations of the patient's condition while focusing only on the positive. For instance, a family may be less understanding and supportive of a patient with a heart attack or alcoholism than the medical condition requires. This may complicate treatment plans ("Oh, it's not serious, Doctor. He just needs to get back in his routine.").

This stage of illness has its own form of ambiguity that makes things difficult. There is uncertainty and unevenness in the pace of recovery, sometimes including sudden shifts in the patient's condition. There are discrepancies in expectations for everyone when the patient does better or worse than predicted. There is a time of marginality when the patient is not clearly an invalid but is not yet fully functioning. Families may not have in their repertoire the ability to make the subtle recalibrations necessary to adjust to these changes or lack of anticipated changes. The more explicit people can be about their expectations, the easier it is to deal with inevitable discrepancies. The health care team can help further by predicting typical setbacks and by normalizing negative feelings that go along with continued upheaval in the family's life. It is also important to note that there is a difference between families who are coping poorly versus families who are coping well with a difficult situation. Well-functioning families themselves are sometimes slow to recognize this distinction and can be encouraged by affirmation from others. They often assume that if they feel sad or discouraged or angry they are coping poorly, yet those feelings are in fact appropriate to the situation they face. They can be assured that it is useful to be aware of those feelings, and that it is not the feelings themselves, but how they act on those feelings that is a better basis for determining how well they are doing.

Deterioration Phase

In the case of terminal illness, family life becomes especially trying. The patient and family are dealing with a whole complex of ultimate issues, and it is exhausting for the family and clinician to deal with a high level of intensity when a patient's illness extends for a long time. However, when someone dies suddenly, family members often suffer from not having had time to reconcile their unfinished business with the patient, besides having little opportunity to make practical adjustments in living without the person. When an illness extends over a long period of time some people feel bad when they fail to have continually intense and "correct" feelings. After long periods of the patient suffering, family members may secretly or overtly wish that the person would die, especially old people who have lived long and well. These feelings seem so toxic, however, that most people can scarcely voice them to themselves, much less to the other family members. Penn (10) referred to "secrets uneasily held" by the patient or family that may include other unacceptable topics such as funeral preparations, life plans for the family after the person is gone, and finances.

Because the family's care of the patient is likely to get more and more difficult for them as a disease progresses, family members face the possibility of becoming totally absorbed in these activities. In a study of end-stage renal patients who were doing home dialysis, Gonzalez and Reiss (12) found that families tended either to neglect other family needs and responsibilities and sacrifice almost everything to care for the patient, or they would minimize their involvement with the illness, leaving the patient to cope alone and trying to operate family life in some normal fashion. Only a rare and exceptional family could manage somehow to meet both sets of needs.

Modern culture's expectations of families are now shifting. Thanks to the advances of medical science and technology, families are expected to take care of people that would never have survived or would have been cared for in an institution in the past. The fact that some patients with very serious illness can be cared for at home is a wonderful thing in some respects. However, the patient's quality of life may be maintained at a tremendous price to the family.

The medical staff who deal with families at the end stage of disease may often be inspired by their courage and closeness. For a time, however, some people have a need *not* to face the full reality of a patient's impending death. It is important for the health care team to view that denial as an active coping strategy on the part of a person who is handling as much as he/she can handle. On the other hand, it may be the health care professionals who struggle to deny impending death, and the family who needs to express acceptance of the end. Allowing a family to mourn may be exceedingly hard for members of the medical team whose training and orientation is toward saving and preserving life. This is another time when feelings and their expression may be out of synchrony in a painful way. As mentioned before, this situation is difficult for mature people at their best. People facing death of a family member are probably exhausted both physically and emotionally, have little privacy, have not been eating well, and have been in strange, technical territory where they are not in control. The tolerance and availability of the health care team can make this situation very good or very bad and may make a difference in how the patient is remembered by the family.

Conclusion

When a patient is ill, a whole set of overlapping processes occurs. The illness itself develops over time, prompting the patient's emotional, functional, and psychological adjustment to it. Family members go through their own processes of adjustment, which may occur at different rates and in different ways. These conditions are superimposed onto ongoing individual and family development, which may make the dependency, discomfort, or trauma of illness especially hard to manage. The patient's circumstances may create more problems in a family that is unable to cope with more complexity.

Families are incredibly resilient, and many strengths will be encountered, some of which the family itself will discover for the first time when they face an illness. For those families who find themselves in an interpersonal crisis, change is always possible and is, in fact, most likely to occur when families are faced with challenges for which their present repertoire of responses seems inadequate. Health care providers can become a significant part of this process that can result in better patient care and rewarding relationships with families.

References

1. Neutra R: Indications for the surgical treatment of suspected acute appendicitis: A cost-effectiveness approach, in Bunker JP, Barnes BA, Mostellar R (eds): Costs, Risks, and Benefits of Surgery. New York, Oxford University Press, 1977.
2. McCubbin HI, Patterson JM: Family stress and adaptation to crises: A double ABCX model of family behavior, in Olson DH, Miller BC (eds): Family Studies Review Yearbook, Vol I. Beverly Hills, CA, Sage, 1983.
3. Hill R: Families under Stress. New York, Harper and Row, 1949.
4. Hoebel FC: Brief family-interactional therapy in the management of cardiac-related high-risk behaviors. J Fam Pract 1976;3:613–618.
5. Oakes TW, Ward JR, Gray RM, Klauber MR, Moody PM: Family expectations and arthritis patient compliance to a hand resting splint regimen. J Chron Dis 1970;22:757–764.
6. Falloon IRH, Boyd JL, McGill CW, Razani J, Moss HB, Gilderman AM: Family management in the prevention of exacerbations of schizophrenia. N Engl J Med 1982;306:1437–1440.
7. Steidl JH, Finkelstein FO, Wexler JP, Feigenbaum H, Kitsen J, Kliger AS, Quinlan DM: Medical conditions, adherence to treatment regimens, and family functioning. Arch Gen Psychiatry 1980;37:1025–1027.
8. Minuchin S, Rosman BL, Baker L: Psychosomatic Families. Cambridge, MA, Harvard University Press, 1978.
9. Tucker S: Family somatics: Of systems, theories and therapy. Paper presented at the 1982 Annual Conference of the American Association of Marital and Family Therapists, Dallas, 1982.
10. Penn P: Families and chronic illness. Paper presented at Ackerman Institute for Family Therapy Conference on Families and Illness, New York, 1982.
11. Speedling E: The Heart Attack. New York, Tavistock Publications, 1982.
12. Gonzales S, Reiss D: The family and chronic illness: Technical difficulties in assessing adjustment. Unpublished paper, Center for Family Research, George Washington University School of Medicine.

CHAPTER 6

Applying a Systems Approach to Common Medical Problems

Thomas Campbell and Susan McDaniel

The clinical application of systems theory to common medical problems can open up new perspectives on diagnosis and new options for treatment of patients and their families. This model, also known as the biopsychosocial model (1), is more than just adding psychosocial data to the biomedical data. A systems approach to health care emphasizes the interdependency and interplay among different levels of the system—whether it is, for example, the interaction among the heart, the cardiovascular system, the individual, significant others, or whether it also includes interactions among factors involving the family, the community, and the society-level systems that can impact health and disease. All interact with one another to affect the patient who walks into a clinic with a presenting complaint. Recognizing and acknowledging the interaction between these different levels of systems allows one to better understand those mysterious, vague, or persistent clinical problems seen in day-by-day practice. The art and science of applying a systems approach to health care turns on the choice of systems levels with which to work. Which areas deserve further exploration and evaluation? Which components might provide the most powerful leverage for successful treatment?

Rather than only describe how a systems approach can be applied to common medical problems, we have chosen to illustrate its use through clinical examples. We will demonstrate how systems theory is relevant to daily clinical practice and need not be overly complex nor take an excessive amount of time. We have drawn cases from our own practices or cases that we have supervised. In each case we will contrast a more traditional "biomedical" approach with a systems or biopsychosocial approach to the problem and then follow the example with a discussion of the important clinical issues raised by the case as well as any research relevant to the problem.

In some of the cases we describe, a systems consultation occurred after an initial biomedial approach was attempted and failed. In other examples, a biopsychosocial approach was tried from the beginning, but we have described a traditional approach to the same problem for point of contrast.

Some of these systems approaches required referral to a specialist for implementation while others required nothing more (and nothing less!) than the physician changing his/her expectations of a patient and family. We recognize that time is of the essence for the practicing clinician. Some of these cases required a greater initial expenditure of time when treated from a systems approach, some required less because fewer tests are run. Overall, we are convinced that a systems approach can reduce the amount of time and expense involved in patient care.

In some cases, a systems approach necessitated the practitioner having greater skill and expertise in working with families. In other cases, the availability of a systems consultation was necessary. Especially in difficult cases, it can be hard for a health care provider to get a clear view of the treatment system that he/she is a part of. Requesting a consultation from one's systems-oriented colleagues can help to clarify diagnosis, treatment, strategy, and any role the provider might play in the presenting problem. Toward this end, we have a group of colleagues who meet weekly to present difficult cases from a systems perspective. In this way, we try to stay current, creative, and flexible in our systems approaches to those difficult, and yet common, medical problems such as diabetes, cardiovascular disease, chronic illness, somatization, depression, and alcoholism.

It would be unfair to present the worst failures of the biomedical approach and to compare them to dramatic successes using a systems approach. The biomedical approach is very successful with many cases, and a systems approach does not always solve the problems. It does, however, open up new options. We have tried to present cases in which excellent traditional medical care was being provided, and then illustrate the advantages a systems approach offers.

Diabetes

A Biomedical Approach to Diabetes

Jim S was a 16-year-old with poorly controlled diabetes. He was first diagnosed as diabetic at the age of 8, when he was admitted to the hospital in a coma secondary to diabetic ketoacidosis (DKA). He initially adapted well to his illness, and by the age of 10 was giving himself his own insulin and generally controlling his own diet. Until the age of 12, he had had only one hospital admission, and that was for a cellulitis of his hand.

At the end of his seventh grade year, Jim's diabetes became more difficult to control. He began consistently spilling large amounts of glucose in his urine, with blood sugars frequently in the 300s. Attempts to increase his insulin led to unpredictable hypoglycemia. Over the next 3 years, Jim had 12 admissions to the hospital for DKA, and two admissions for hypoglycemia. While in the hospital each time, his blood sugars were easily controlled on lower doses of insulin than what he had been on at home. He stated that he was sticking to his diet and denied any snacking or drinking alcohol. In this period, his behavior at home and at school had become a problem as well. He would refuse to do any household chores and got in frequent fights with his stepfather, which were at times physical. His mother and stepfather were at their wits' ends. They felt they could no longer control his behavior, or assure that he took his insulin properly. They were worried about his poorly controlled diabetes and frequent infections. They turned to his physician for help.

The physician became very involved in this case and sought to get Jim to take more control of his illness. She encouraged him to measure his own blood glucose at home and adjust his own insulin. She discouraged the parents' supervision of his diabetes. Unfortunately, he would "forget" to bring in the records of his blood sugars, and frequently missed appointments. The physician alternated between being understanding with Jim, feeling the parents were to blame for being so intrusive, and being very angry with the boy for not taking care of himself. After three hospitalizations over a 2-month period, the parents said they could not handle him any longer, and requested that the physician hospitalize him for a more extended period of time to "really get his diabetes under control."

Insulin-dependent diabetes mellitus (IDDM) is a chronic illness that often begins in childhood or adolescence and requires major changes in the lives of patients and their families. Tight metabolic control of blood sugar appears to prevent some of the complications of the illness (nephropathy, retinopathy, and neuropathy). Optimal management of the illness requires careful regulation of diet, exercise, and insulin dosages. Many programs expect diabetics to check their own blood sugars (by finger stick) three to five times a day, and to give themselves insulin two or more times a day. The functioning of the family and the psychosocial adjustment of the diabetic will affect the ability to adhere to such a complex and regimented program.

Unfortunately, IDDM is too often considered merely a disorder of carbohydrate metabolism, and, as in this case, a biomedical solution (more insulin and stricter diet) is applied to a biopsychosocial problem. In managing diabetes, at least four systemic levels must be attended to: the physiologic (i.e., glucose regulation); the individual (i.e., psychological development); the family (i.e., response to illness); and larger social systems (e.g., health care system, school, peers). The biomedical approach outlined above considers only the first two levels of the system (physiologic and individual). Inadequate attention is paid to the social context of the illness and the interactions between the diabetic, the family, and the physician.

In this case, as is common in clinical practice, very little psychosocial information or history about the patient and his family was obtained. In the past, physicians have been better trained and more skilled in the management of insulin dosages than in assessing and working with families. Recurrent "biomedical crises" divert attention away from psychosocial assessment to the urgent control of the diabetes. The family in this case example also viewed the primary problem as a biomedical one. Feeling helpless, they requested that the biomedical expert take charge of the problem and hospitalize their son. The physician repeated the same pattern as the parents, reasoning with the adolescent and encouraging him to become more independent and take more responsibility for his illness, but without success. Both the parents and the physician were frustrated and felt helpless. They appeared more worried about the diabetes than the patient, who asserted his autonomy from the family and the health care providers by keeping only marginal control of his diabetes. To take a biopsychosocial or systems view of the problem requires that the physician step back out of the system of which he/she is a part and, in this case, seek consultation.

A Biopsychosocial Approach to Diabetes

At the point of hospitalization, the family physician requested a consult from a group of colleagues interested in biopsychosocial medicine and the role of families in illness and treatment. This consultation resulted in the following treatment strategies:

1. Gather more information about the family and their responses to Jim's diabetes.
2. Use the hospitalization to stabilize Jim and bring some organization and structure to the chaos and stress in the family.
3. Use the parents, especially, as resources and authorities who can help Jim to treat his diabetes appropriately when he is irresponsible about it.
4. When Jim takes good care of himself and handles his diabetes appropriately, he earns autonomy and adult status (i.e., more freedom). His parents may only intrude when Jim is "immature" and irresponsible about his diabetes.
5. Consult with a family therapist to hold joint family sessions during the hospitalization.
6. Discharge only when the physician, patient, and family meet all the above goals.

When the physician took a family history from Jim's parents, she found that this was a multiproblem family with multiple stressors over the past several years (see Figure 6.1). Jim's diabetes was only one of many problems with which this family had to cope. The physician discovered Mr. and Mrs. S had had an unplanned pregnancy, followed closely by Mr. S losing his job and then Mrs. S developing multiple pregnancy-related medical problems. Soon after the baby was born, the family home burned to the ground. The family then moved three times over the next 6 months. The public health nurse sent out to check on the baby literally could not find this family. In this same time period, Jim drifted through three different schools, though his attendance at any of them was sporadic at best. Under considerable strain, Mr. and Mrs. S were quite worried about their children's many problems, especially Jim's diabetes, but were unable to set limits or provide appropriate guidance in most situations; hence, the strategy to use the hospitalization to both stabilize Jim's diabetes and stabilize and structure his family environment. Without the latter, a systems approach would predict a strong likelihood that hospitalization would bring temporary symptomatic relief, only to send Jim out to an environment in which he would again be careless with his disease.

Using the hospitalization as a convenient time for a family gathering, the physician, a family therapist, and the nurse practitioner most involved in Jim's outpatient treatment met with all the members of Jim's household to implement strategies 3 and 4. To accomplish these goals, the family therapist, with the support of the medical team, urged Mr. and Mrs. S to supervise Jim's care of his diabetes.

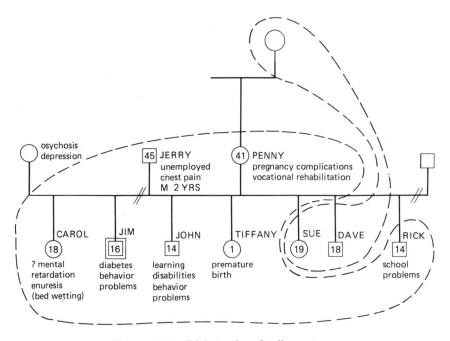

FIGURE 6.1.   Diabetes in a family system.

The parents formulated a plan in the first session to check Jim's compliance, allowing him freedom when he complied and restricting his freedom and managing his disease themselves when he did not. Here the family therapist and the physician underlined the parents' authority while still supporting Jim's need for independence when he handled himself responsibly. Jim was discharged after this session, the treatment goals having been achieved.

After discharge, this same treatment team met with the family on three more occasions to monitor this new plan and to support the new family organization. As with many medical problems, it was an essential part of this systems strategy for the physician to conceptualize and work with the important members of the treatment system: the family, the hospital staff, the family therapist, the school, etc. While this approach did not magically resolve all this family's many problems, it did succeed in stabilizing Jim's diabetes, increasing his healthy autonomy in the family, and providing a model for the parents to problem solve with their children. It also channeled the physician's frustration and concern into a clear and organized treatment plan.

Salvador Minuchin, a leader in the field of family therapy, worked with the families of children with chronic illnesses at the Philadelphia Child Guidance Clinic (2,3). He found that many of the diabetic children improved dramatically on lower doses of insulin when admitted to the hospital, but upon returning home their diabetes worsened. He studied intensively the families of children with brittle diabetes, stress-induced asthma, and anorexia nervosa and found common patterns of interaction.

The children were all involved in parental conflict. ~~~ they were in a *coalition* with one parent against another or the con~~~ was detoured through the child. The families' structure was characterized by: (a) enmeshment—family members overreacting to the stress of another member and demonstrating a lack of autonomy; (b) overprotectiveness—family members not being allowed to handle their own problems individually; (c) rigidity—transactional patterns are repeated inflexibly, and change is resisted; and (d) conflict avoidance—the open airing of disagreement is not permitted and problems are not resolved. These family characteristics tended to worsen the child's symptoms, and the symptoms prevented any resolution of the parent's conflicts and preserved the rigidity.

Minuchin called these families "psychosomatic families," because the family interactions have a direct effect on the child's illness. He studied changes in free fatty acid (FFA) levels in the diabetic children during stressful family interviews (4,5). The psychosomatic diabetics had a marked rise in their FFA level while they were observing a family conflict through a one-way mirror. The FFAs rose further when the child was brought into the conflict, while the FFAs of the mother decreased simultaneously. These changes were not observed in the families of non-psychosomatic diabetics. Minuchin hypothesized that the child's level of stress was leading to increased blood sugar and FFAs and eventually diabetic ketoacidosis.

Minuchin and his colleagues treated a group of these children with severe diabetes, asthma, and anorexia nervosa, using structural family therapy (2). Treatments lasted 4–12 months and were designed to change the psychosomatic structures of the families. Repeated patterns of recurrent hospitalizations, chronic ketonuria in the diabetics, and steroid dependence in the asthmatics virtually disappeared. Medication use in the asthmatics and insulin dosages were drastically reduced. All the anorectics recovered, with weight gains of 5–30 pounds over 1–4 years.

Minuchin's work with psychosomatic families is a landmark for the application of systems theory in chronic illness. However, there are several problems with his approach. The term "psychosomatic" is a poor one in that it carries connotations associated with the early research in psychosomatic medicine. To many, it implies that these illness are not as "real" or "organic" as other illnesses, or that other illnesses are not psychosomatic. It is better to think of all families as psychosomatic, just as all illnesses are psychosomatic; that is, family and psychological processes can affect the course or development of any illness.

The work by Minuchin suggests that certain family characteristics are specific for families of poorly controlled diabetics, asthmatics, and anorectics. Yet, there have been very few controlled studies of the families of ill children. These characteristics (enmeshment, overprotectiveness, rigidity, conflict avoidance) may be common in families with any type of chronic illness. Furthermore, other studies of diabetic children suggest that poor control of blood sugar is due to a combination of lack of compliance and a direct physiologic effect that mediates the effect of family factors on diabetic control (6,7).

Cardiovascular Disease

A Biomedical Approach to Cardiovascular Disease

Mrs. Jones, a 30-year-old woman, telephoned her physician about her 42-year-old husband. She was concerned that Mr. Jones was going to have a heart attack. He was a moderately successful executive in a high pressure job, and was on the road for many weeks of the year. Over the past few months, the business had been having financial problems, for which, according to the wife, the husband felt responsible. He had not been sleeping at night and was so preoccupied by his work that he had ceased paying any attention to their 6-month-old son. He smoked 1–2 packs of cigarettes a day and did not exercise. The husband's father died of a heart attack at the age of 45. The wife did not know whether her husband was having any chest pain, but was certain that he would not tell her if he had. The physician had met the husband during the wife's pregnancy, but had never been consulted for any health concerns.

Based upon the information provided by the wife, the physician wrote the husband a letter suggesting that he come in for a "routine physical examination," which the husband agreed to. During the visit, the husband admitted he was under a great deal of stress and smoked too much, but he said he was working on both problems. He denied any cardiac symptoms. While he expressed some concern about his family history of heart disease, he felt he was in "pretty good shape." He did express some annoyance over his wife's nagging him about his work and health, and admitted that he came in for the physical to "get her off my back." His physical exam was unremarkable except for mild obesity. His electrocardiogram and spirometry (measure of lung function) were normal and his cholesterol was mildly elevated (235). The patient underwent an exercise tolerance test (stress test), which was also normal.

The physician strongly recommended that the patient stop smoking completely, prescribed nicotine gum, and gave him the names of several local smoking cessation programs. In addition, the physician outlined an exercise program and referred him to the practice's dietician for a low cholesterol diet. The physician offered to teach him some relaxation techniques to deal with stress, but the patient declined, saying he could best deal with the stress on his own. A follow-up appointment was made for 3 months later, which the patient later cancelled. The wife informed the physician that her husband had not followed any of his instructions and that nothing had changed, except that the couple was arguing more about the husband's health. When the physician called the husband, he refused to come in again, saying that he did not see any need for it.

Coronary heart disease (CHD) remains the leading cause of death in the United States. The risk factors for CHD (smoking, hypertension, lack of exercise, diabetes, hypercholesterolemia, family history of CHD, Type A personality) are well understood, and, except for family history, can be modified. While the treatment of hypertension is relatively easy, most clinicians find it very difficult and often frustrating to get patients to change their life-style: to stop smoking, eat fewer calories and less cholesterol, exercise more, and reduce stress.

This case example represents an excellent medical and individual approach to preventive cardiology. Several risk factors were identified and specific interventions were attempted. The physician was aware of the latest approaches to risk reduction (nicotine gum, low cholesterol diet, exercise programs, and relaxation techniques). However, in this case the approach did not work, and the interventions were not successful, partly because the broader context of the problem was not considered. The wife's initial phone call should suggest to the physician that these behaviors play an important role in the couple's relationship. A physician using a systems approach might handle this problem in a different way.

A Systems Approach to Cardiovascular Disease

After listening to the concerns of Mrs. Jones about her husband, Dr. C thanked her for the valuable information, commenting that her perspective on her husband's behavior and health was very important. He suggested that she should join her husband when he comes in for a physical exam so that a more complete picture of the problem can be obtained. In addition, Dr. C said he wanted to hear what suggestions she might have for helping her husband. Dr. C instructed her to tell her husband everything that they had discussed on the phone, and that he was recommending that he come in with his wife to discuss these concerns. Dr. C offered to talk with the husband prior to the visit. Despite some reluctance on Mr. Jones' part, Mrs. Jones did accompany her husband for the doctor's visit.

Dr. C spent the beginning of the session listening to the concerns of each member of the couple. The wife reiterated her fears about her husband's health, but emphasized the stress of his job and the time he was spending away from home. Mr. Jones said he was concerned about his health, but resented his wife's nagging about it. He felt he could change on his own and would not follow his wife's advice. After some discussion, it became clear that the husband's health was a small part of larger marital conflict. Mrs. Jones wanted her husband to help more around the house and with their child. She was furious that they had not had sex since their baby's birth. Mr. Jones felt excluded from the mother–child relationship and was experiencing increasing financial burdens with the new family member. While their relationship had been quite good prior to the pregnancy, they had been fighting frequently since the birth of the new baby.

After further discussion, the couple agreed that both of them had health problems (the wife had menstrual irregularities), but that each should take responsibility for his/her own problems. In particular, the wife agreed not to make suggestions about her husband's health unless he asked for them. The husband agreed to have a complete physical examination, and to begin to make some changes in his life-style. Dr. C told them that their relationship appeared to be under increased stress since the arrival of the baby, but that this was quite common after the birth of a first child. He suggested that they come in together again in several weeks to see how the agreement about health problems was working, and to assist them in reducing the stress if they so desired.

In the first approach to this problem, the physician accepted the wife's description of her husband's problem at face value, and unwittingly joined her in a coalition against the husband. This actually weakened the physician's influence with the husband, for he viewed the physician as an agent of his wife. Family members commonly tell their family physician about other members of the family, and sometimes ask that the conversation be kept in confidence. The physician must be extremely cautious that he/she not be pulled into the family conflict. He/she should avoid listening to one side of the story over the phone, or agreeing to keep secrets in confidence.

In the systems approach to the problem, the physician recognized that there was some conflict between the couple about the husband's health and that the wife was displaying more concern than her husband about his health. Dr. C was aware that the wife was trying to get him to join in her crusade to change her husband. He assumed that the husband was concerned about his own health, but hypothesized that his wife's approach might result in his resisting any change. The crucial step in this approach was to invite both members of the couple in together, so that the wife could express her concerns directly to the husband and not through the physician. The physician could maintain an alliance with both of them and explore the problem in more depth.

Knowledge of the family life cycle and the tasks that individual patients and their families face is extremely helpful in the understanding and treatment of many problems seen in the physician's office (see Chapter 4). In this case, the problems were part of the process of moving from a two-person marital system to a three-person family, with new parental roles and responsibilities. This family was having some difficulty negotiating this stage; their difficulties led to marital conflict and then presented to the physician as health concerns.

The relationship between the physician, patient, and family is best viewed as a triad or therapeutic triangle (8). Within any triad, there is a tendency for two in the system to join in a coalition against the third. Most commonly, this is the physician and the patient blaming another family member (e.g., an inattentive husband or authoritarian parents) for the patient's problems. In this case, it was a family member, the wife, who wants the physician on her side. To be effective in changing dysfunctional systems, the physician must avoid *coalitions* (two against one), but maintain *alliances* with both the family and the patient.

Studies of the role of the family in compliance suggest that the family can be a powerful therapeutically. Morisky and colleagues at Johns Hopkins used a randomized controlled trial to study the impact of family involvement on hypertension over a 5-year period (9). A survey indicated that 70% of their hypertensive patients expressed a desire for their families to learn more about their illness. Several groups of patients received a home visit during which a family member (usually the spouse) was educated about hypertension. When compared to the control group, these patients had fewer missed appointments, better blood pressure control, and a 57% decrease in overall mortality. Hoebel worked with the wives of "difficult cardiac patients" who would not change their risk factors (smoking, diet, lack of exercise, and Type A behavior) (10). He showed the women how their own behaviors were maintaining the high risk behaviors of their husbands, and taught them what they could do to modify those behaviors. With only the spouses being seen, seven of nine cardiac patients changed their high risk behaviors.

The best known research on the family and heart disease comes from the Israel Ischemic Heart Disease Project, a prospective study similar to the Framingham Study. Medalie and colleagues followed 10,000 civil servants over 5 years for the development of heart disease, and found that family problems were as strong a predictor for the development of angina as any physiologic variable, including blood pressure, cholesterol levels, and the electrocardiogram (11). Furthermore, in men with high anxiety, "wife's love and support" protected against the development of angina (12). It did not affect men with low anxiety, suggesting a buffering effect of family support.

Several studies have shown a relationship between family support and compliance with different therapeutic regimens (13–15). As part of a trial of a cholestrol lowering agent, Doherty was able to demonstrate a correlation between specific behaviors of the wife and compliance by the husband with the medication (16). These behaviors included "showing interest in the program" and "reminding him about his medicine and diet." "Nagging about his medicine or diet" was negatively correlated with compliance. The wife's health beliefs regarding the benefits of treatment and the husband's susceptibility to the risks of elevated cholesterol correlated with her support.

Doherty and Baird have developed a protocol for involving families in compliance counseling (17). They recommended the following procedures in such cases. Convene the family whenever adherence to a medical regimen is likely to be difficult. Begin with a discussion of the medical problem and elicit questions and reactions from the family. Encourage the family to express their feelings about the patient's illness and the treatment plan. Then assist the patient and his/her family to negotiate what kind of assistance can be given and is desired by the patient. By the end of such a session, there should be a behavioral contract in which the family agrees to provide support without being intrusive. Finally, schedule a follow-up session to assess how effective the family's support is in promoting compliance.

Chronic Illness

A Biomedical Approach to a Family With Multiple Chronic Illnesses

The Bunker family did not like visiting physicians (see Figure 6.2). Mrs. Bunker was 61 years old and had severe chronic obstructive pulmonary disease (COPD) due to smoking. She had been hospitalized numerous times and had to be placed on a respirator on two occasions. She has oxygen at home which she used at

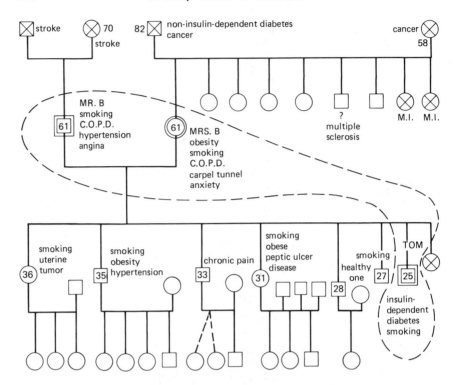

FIGURE 6.2. Multiple chronic illnesses in a family system.

night. She complained of intermittent chest pain, due to gastritis and esophageal reflux. She also had bilateral carpal tunnel syndrome, but refused surgery. She continued to smoke a pack of cigarettes per day (reduced from two), and took Librium three times a day for anxiety.

Mr. Bunker was a 61-year-old electrician. He had hypertension, mild COPD, and chronic stable angina. He smoked 1½ packs of cigarettes a day. He was unable to take nitrates for his angina because of headaches, and beta blockers worsened his lung disease. Despite adjustments in his medication, he usually had several episodes of chest pain per week. He had difficulty making office appointments due to his demanding job, and frequently requested refills of his medication over the phone. When he did see his physician, Dr. T, he expressed concern about his health and a willingness to do whatever his physician requested.

Tom Bunker was the youngest son and the only child living at home with his parents. He was 25 and unemployed. He has been an insulin-dependent diabetic for 12 years. He checked his blood sugars at home two to three times a day and adjusted his own insulin. He kept a diary of his insulin and blood sugars, and it indicated that his diabetes was in good control. However, when he was seen in the office, his blood sugars were very high (250–350) and his glycosylated hemoglobin level (a measure of chronic control) was also elevated. A diet history revealed that he was knowledgeable about the diabetic diet, and he said he stuck to it fairly closely. He smoked 2 packs of cigarettes a day, and had tried to stop on numerous occasions without success.

Dr. T found this family both pleasant and frustrating to deal with. They came for appointments only when they needed refills on their medication. They were very concerned about each other's health, and would talk about how important it was for one of the others to come in to be checked. Each of them recited how bad smoking is, and how much they wanted to quit. Several attempts to quit as a family had been unsuccessful. Their family physician had come to feel powerless, and tended to refill their medications over the phone, extending the intervals between visits even further.

Most of physicians' training occurs within the hospital, and involves the treatment of acute illness or exacerbations of chronic illness. Many physicians find curing disease more satisfying than managing chronic illness. Therefore, they may be unprepared to care for patients in their practices with chronic illnesses, which cannot be cured and may not improve. While physicians may treat acute illnesses, they help patients manage their chronic illness. Thus, management of chronic disease includes not only proper use of medication and dietary and activity changes, but assisting patients in adapting to their limitations.

Caring for patients with chronic illnesses can be time consuming and exhausting. Caring for families with multiple chronic illnesses can be overwhelming. One common pitfall for physicians is trying to take charge of the illness, and impose one's own goals onto the patient. Often physicians do not appreciate the role that chronic illness plays in the patient's life and in the family. In this case, the son will not care for his diabetes, so that the parents can continue to worry about their youngest child and take care of him, and do not have to face the empty nest and reestablishing their marital relationship. Efforts to get the son to be more responsible without considering the effects on the family are not likely to be successful.

Chronic illness can provoke a power struggle between the physician and patient. The physician may feel responsible for the health of his/her patient, believing that it reflects on the quality of his/her care. The physician wants his/her patients to "take better care of themselves," to stop smoking, lose weight, or keep better control of their blood sugars. The more severe the chronic illness, the more responsible the physician may feel for changing these behaviors. On the other hand, patients have different priorities and different needs. The illness may be tightly interwoven into the fabric of family interactions. Many patients are unwilling or unable to give up smoking, lose weight, or maintain tighter diabetic control. Rather than negotiating a compromise, the physician and patient fight over control of the illness, sometimes overtly, but usually covertly, as in the case example. However, the physician cannot win since it is not his/her illness, and such an approach leads to dissatisfaction on the parts of both the patient and physician and to poor health care.

A Systems Approach to Chronic Illnesses

Systems thinking offers a different approach to chronic illness. Chronic illness, by definition, is stable, and becomes part of the day-to-day experience of family life. With the Bunkers, multiple chronic illnesses were integral to the identity (for better or worse) of this family. Family members were caught up, quite literally, in a vicious repetitive pattern in which each worried about the other while being both irresponsible and hopeless about his/her own behavior. Family member A said to family member B: "I cannot change, but you have to change because you are so sick." Family member B said to family member A: "I cannot change, but you have to change because you are so sick." Widening our perspective from the family system to the physician–family system, the family repeatedly said to the physician: "I cannot be helped because I will not do what I need to do to help myself—my situation is impossible and hopeless, but you must help my mother/father/son. Meanwhile, I will be a polite patient and pretend to accept your suggestions and do what is necessary." The physician repeatedly made good suggestions to the family and felt frustrated by their lack of compliance. He was inducted into the family in the sense that he shared their hopelessness and frustration about others not changing.

Having diagnosed the problems from a systems point of view, Dr. T. chose to pursue the following strategies. First, recognizing that the repetitive theme was that everyone waits for someone else to change first, he decided to be the first person in the treatment system to change his own behavior, stop "smoking," so to speak, and do something different, completely independent of whether it produces change for anyone else (i.e., the family).

Second, Dr. T decided to use his time differently: rather than treating this family P.R.N. and for medications, he set up regular meetings with each of them. To begin with, he convened a family meeting to discuss everyone's current health status, discuss their concern for each other, how they had been unable to change despite good intentions, and his sadness about that. He told the family he needed to have family meetings like that every 6 months because they had so many chronic illnesses among them, they needed to be kept informed about each other, and it was the most cost-effective and efficient way to manage their treatment. Given the likely outcome to many of these problems, he knew these meetings were a necessity for them all to be able to work together, physician and family, to deal with the problems ahead.

Third, in shifting the way he had thought about this family, Dr. T had become more and more curious about them, realizing they had a lot to teach him. For this family who had learned how to appear healthy while actually being quite sick, the risk of truly changing must have been great indeed. (For example, Mr. Bunker may have feared that if he stopped smoking he would become more nervous, yell more at his wife who he felt could not take it, and even precipitate a massive heart attack in himself.) Dr. T decided to spend his individual and family sessions trying to understand what must have been powerful risks for the Bunker family members in changing their behavior.

Finally, given the chronicity and duration of the symptoms, Dr. T listed two very small realistic goals for treatment over the next year for each family member and for himself as provider:

Dr. T:
1. To understand better the risk of change for this family.
2. To stay connected through structured appointments without needed the family members to be healthy.

Mr. Bunker:
1. To come in every 4 months (rather than every 6 months).
2. To have Mrs. Bunker accompany him to appointments (to provide more information about the angina and potentially increase compliance).
Mrs. Bunker:
1. To come in every 2 months for an office visit (rather than every 4 months).
2. To consult a neurosurgeon for her carpal tunnel syndrome.
Tommy Bunker:
1. To come in every month for 4 months.
2. To keep a diary of daily blood sugars, and bring it in with the chemistry sticks used to measure the blood sugars.

The Ackerman Institute for Family Therapy's Chronic Illness Project has found that families coping with chronic illness, such as the Bunkers, can have two common characteristics: dysfunctional cross-generational coalitions that stabilize due to the illness (e.g., an overly close relationship between mother and son becomes acceptable or even prescribed when he becomes sick) and stagnation or "stuckness" in terms of emotional development when the family cannot move beyond the stage they were in when the illness first became problematic (18, 19). Unlike families with psychiatric illness such as schizophrenia or anorexia nervosa, these families do not hide or deny these coalitions, but accept them openly as a consequence of the illness.

Often these family interactions recapitulate cross-generational coalitions from the parents' families of origin. What may initially have been a functional adaptation becomes rigid and resistant to change, even when the illness improves or resolves completely. Penn has suggested that, in addition to obtaining the genogram of families with chronic illness, the health care provider should ask what each family member's explanation and expectation of the illness is (18). This information will give the physician a better understanding of what role the illness plays in the family. With the Bunker family, it was unclear how relational patterns might affect family members' illnesses. A family meeting to gather such information was an important next step. One might hypothesize that, given the family's stage in the life cycle, one problem may involve Tom's attempts as the youngest child to leave home and become an independent adult. Addressing the full range of biopsychosocial issues in this case may help to better understand the meaning of these illnesses to the family, increase compliance, and eventually encourage overall health for all family members.

Somatization

A Biomedical Approach to Somatization

The Peace family had been patients of Dr. M for several years. The children, ages 7 and 4, had been seen for numerous office visits, mostly with viral illnesses. The older child, Shawn, had had repeated episodes of sore throat and tonsilitis, missing several weeks of school each year. Although throat cultures for streptococcus had always been negative, he was eventually referred to an otolaryngologist at the mother's request and had a tonsillectomy. Terry, the younger child, has had recurrent ear infections, and recently had tympanostomy tubes inserted into each ear.

Shortly after Terry's tube insertions, Mrs. Peace came to Dr. M for a complete physical, and complained of crampy abdominal pain and intermittent diarrhea. Her examination was unremarkable except for a 4–5-cm adnexal mass felt on pelvic exam, which appeared cystic on ultrasound. She was treated with mild analgesics for a presumed ovarian cyst. The pain worsened over the next week, and then disappeared, as did the cyst. However, the diarrhea persisted for another month, and increased to the extent that Mrs. Peace could not leave her house for fear of being distant from a bathroom. An extensive gastrointestinal work-up, including stool cultures, upper gastrointestinal series, barium enema, sigmoidoscopy, and studies for malabsorption were all normal. Dr. M prescribed a high fiber diet and antidiarrhea medication, which lessened the symptoms.

As Mrs. Peace's diarrhea was gradually improving, Mr. Peace consulted Dr. M for the first time. He complained of a persistent low back pain, which he said was interfering with his farming. On examination, his prostate was mildly tender, and his urinalysis revealed 1–2 white cells per high powered field. His urine culture was negative, but he was treated with antibiotics for a presumed prostatitis. While on antibiotics, he developed left testicular pain, and noticed a bluish discoloration of his scrotum. Examinations by Dr. M and a consulting urologist were unremarkable. His pains decreased after prolonged antibiotic therapy, but did not completely resolve.

Over the next 6 months, Dr. M saw either Mr. or Mrs. Peace every 2 to 3 weeks. During that time, Mrs. Peace also reported some low back pain that radiated down her right leg. She was briefly admitted to the hospital when she developed weakness of both legs and urinary retention. Her evaluation included back X-rays, computerized tomography, and tests for multiple sclerosis, all of which were negative. Her urinary retention resolved without treatment, and she was discharged. However, she continued to complain of leg weakness and back pain, and insisted to Dr. M that there had to be something wrong and that she should have further tests.

Patients with multiple somatic complaints for which no physiologic explanation can be found are commonly seen in clinical practice and are some of the most difficult and frustrating patients for a physician to work with. They present with complaints that range from seemingly trivial (frequent colds), to those that are easy to diagnose but difficult to treat (headaches, chronic back pain), to complex and very worrisome symptoms (lower extremity weakness). These patients are very somatically focused, often insisting on more and more tests to find out "what is wrong" with them. Reassurance is rarely helpful. They are resistant to psychosocial exploration, and may accuse the physician of suggesting the symptoms are "not real" and that "it's all in their heads." For these reasons, such patients often refuse referrals to mental health professionals, and when psychiatrists do see these patients they report little success with them.

The typical approach with these patients is to begin with diagnosis by exclusion. Possible medical illnesses that might produce the symptoms are "ruled out," and the physician tries to reassure the patient that nothing serious is wrong. When everything physiologic has been excluded, and the symptoms persist or new perplexing symptoms develop, the physician may begin to explore psychosocial factors. Usually the patient insists that everything is fine, except for his/her symptoms. The physician feels powerless and frustrated, and attempts to reduce contact with the patient. These patients are often labeled with a psychiatric diagnosis, such as hypochondriasis, hysteria, somatoform disorder, Briquet's syndrome, or depression. Unfortunately, with the exception of depression, these diagnoses rarely help in the management of these patients. It is often better to avoid specific labeling, and use the concept of somatization, a process in which psychologic states are expressed through bodily symptoms.

Family physicians have an advantage in the treatment of somatization because it commonly involves the entire family. Pediatricians see children who are brought in repeatedly by parents for minor concerns or illnesses. They may not know that the mother frequently sees her gynecologist for persistent vaginal discharge or pelvic pain, or that the husband is out of work because of low back pain. A family physician has an opportunity to work with the entire family and understand the role of the somatic symptoms in the family. In order to understand and manage these disorders, one needs to use a systems approach, which may include not only the family but also the work or school system, utilizing the multiple resources within the community.

A Systems Approach to Somatization

The treatment and management of the Peace family was filled with mystery, challenge, and frustration for Dr. M (and for the family). Dr. M clearly had established some minor findings with each of these patients, but not nearly enough to explain their various, and at times severe, aches and pains. Clearly, the traditional biomedical approach was not sufficient for these patients.

Slowly, Dr. M began gathering bits and pieces of family history. At first, both Mr. and Mrs. Peace reported pleasant childhoods and a happy family life now. Gradually, contradictory information began to surface as Mrs. Peace especially began to open up more and more (see Figure 6.3). From her, Dr. M learned that, at 16, Mr. Peace had been abandoned by his parents and left in a cabin on top of a hill with his five younger siblings, forced to work and take care of them at an early age. Mrs. Peace said she, herself, had been somewhat estranged from her own mother, who was now dead; she also implied in a roundabout way that she was now experiencing some marital discord.

With these hints and the persistent vague complaints from both patients, Dr. M suggested an evaluation session with a family therapist to explore the role of stress in each of their chronic somatic problems.

At this session, Dr. M and Dr. S, the family therapist, tried to widen the perspective on these somatically focused patients' problems. Through careful questioning, they learned of the intense work schedules both of these people had kept before becoming sick, rising at 4 AM and doing hard manual labor until after sundown to keep their farm going. Their aches and pains seemed to alternate, so that

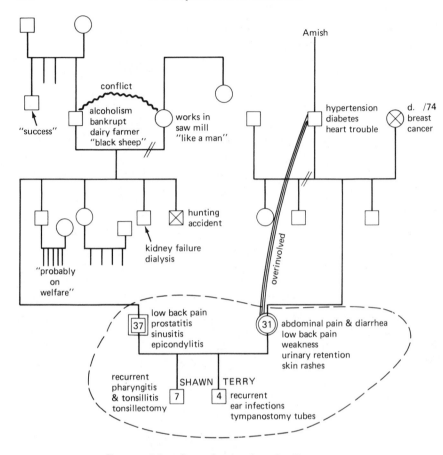

FIGURE 6.3. Somatization in a family system.

at no time were both patients out of commission and the farm unattended. As more focused questions were asked about family of origin issues by the family therapist, it became clear that the couple was quite anxious about these matters. Mrs. Peace became more withdrawn and Mr. Peace excluded some areas of inquiry he felt would be "too much" for his wife. Later in the session, the ice seemed to be broken when Mr. Peace told the story of his childhood abandonment, a story he claimed he never shared with others except his wife. Without overwhelming this couple, both Dr. M and Dr. S felt this session was successful in focusing treatment on the pain in the Peaces' families as well in their backs. It was agreed, at the end of the session, that the couple would begin family therapy with Dr. S, that Dr. M would continue to manage the treatment of Mr. and Mrs. Peace, and that Drs. M and S would collaborate to provide the most comprehensive multisystems approach to this complicated family.

Over time, many family secrets emerged in both Dr. M's and Dr. S's offices, such as Mrs. Peace's abuse as a child, her marrying against her parents' wishes, and her guilt over her mother's sudden death soon after her marriage. Relaxation exercises, psychotherapy, and restructuring of the family life-style began paying off with diminished physical symptoms in both patients. Over a year's period, these patients each got in touch with anger toward their parents, worked the anger through, and reconnected with their families in a more healthy way. (Mr. Peace began visiting his mother after refusing to see her for 15 years.) Mrs. Peace 'reconciled' with her mother through frequent trips to the mother's gravesite, where she was able to confront some painful issues. Throughout the experience, Mr. and Mrs. Peace had to deal with some difficult sexual issues as well as learning to express anger with each other in a healthy way. Mrs. Peace reported working hard to teach her children to be honest and expressive "so they don't have to go through the same thing."

Throughout the year and a half of family therapy, Drs. M and S worked hard to coordinate and dovetail their treatment plans for this family, allowing an integration of the somatic and psychologic components experienced by various members of the Peace family. Mrs. Peace continued to see Dr. M for various difficult, but responsive, pains and skin rashes. Mr. Peace was seen by Dr. M episodically for prostatitis, sinusitis, and occupation-related epicondylitis. What had been unmanageable became manageable.

Patients who frequently express themselves through somatic complaints can be expensive, requiring both time and money. When Mr. and Mrs. Peace first became symptomatic, their problems seemed mysterious and frustrating for the physician. He performed the appropriate diagnostic tests with no positive results. He became somatically fixated himself, performing more and more tests, determined to find the cause of these symptoms. Shifting gears and taking a systems approach, and then collaborating with a family therapist, allowed this difficult family to become interesting and workable. Dr. M found he could tolerate the uncertainty inherent in this family and focus on helping them to feel better. This family will probably always be relatively heavy utilizers of health care services, but their pain and frustration have radically diminished, and they have developed the ability to enjoy their lives and overcome the chronic depression that had plagued each of them for many years.

Van Eijk, Huygens, and their colleagues in the Netherlands have studied the process of "somatic fixation" in patients and believe that the family doctor plays a critical role in this process (20). They view "somatic fixation . . . as a result of continuous one-sided emphasis on the somatic aspects of diseases, complaints, or problem"—in other words, the biomedical approach. To prevent somatic fixation, the authors believe that the physician must be able to integrate the psychosocial and somatic aspects of care, be alert to signals of psychologic distress (such as recent stressful life events), and appropriately share with the patient the responsibility for alleviating the symptom.

Doherty and Baird suggested a number of strategies for redefining somatic symptoms in biopsychosocial terms (8):

1. Allow time for nonfocused, open-ended questions.
2. Introduce psychosocial issues while evaluating medical symptoms.

3. Assure the patient that you are conducting an appropriately thorough medical evaluation.
4. Avoid premature reassurances about benign complaints.
5. When complaints are serious, do not lose sight of the family implications.
6. Stay involved with the family after a referral.
7. Bide your time when your first attempt does not work.
8. Make a strong confrontation with patients who are in serious psychosocial difficulty.
9. Avoid perfunctory questions such as, "How's the marriage (or sex life)?", and blunt statements such as, "I can find nothing physically wrong, so it must be mental" or "I think your family is part of the problem."

Depression

A Biomedical Approach to Depression

Mr. Kalish is a 58-year-old schoolteacher, who presented to his family physician, Dr. E, complaining of fatigue and weight loss. He had been in good health, but over the previous 3 months had noted the gradual onset of generalized malaise and loss of appetite, without nausea or vomiting. He was having increasing difficulty concentrating on his work, and felt exhausted by midday. Despite the fatigue, he slept poorly and awoke frequently throughout the night. The rest of his review of symptoms was unremarkable. He reported a family history of depression in his maternal grandmother.

A more detailed history revealed that the symptoms had begun shortly after the patient had lost a large sum of money in a bad investment, and that he had had a similar episode several years before. At that time, the symptoms resolved after several months without seeking treatment. This time, he had attempted to build up his strength and endurance with exercises and vitamins, but they only seemed to make him feel more fatigued. He was particularly concerned that he might lose his job because of his illness. He denied suicidal ideation.

Mr. Kalish's physical examination was unremarkable except for a depressed affect and a 15-pound weight loss since the previous visit 6 months ago. Screening laboratory tests (complete blood count, routine chemistries, and thyroid function tests) were also normal. A dexamethasone suppression test (DST) was performed and was abnormal (failed to suppress), suggesting depression.

Dr. E started the patient on amitryptyline, a tricyclic antidepressant, and gradually increased the medication up to the maximum dose over 6 weeks. The sleeping difficulties improved promptly and his appetite increased. After 3 months on the maximum dose, Mr. Kalish felt better, having more energy and a slight increase in his weight. However, he continued to have difficulty concentrating, and remained very concerned about his health and his job. An amitryptyline level was checked and was in the therapeutic range. A repeat DST was now normal. Dr. E recommended individual counseling as a supplement to the medication, and referred Mr. Kalish to a psychodynamically oriented psychotherapist. Mr. Kalish experienced some improvement during treatment, which involved weekly sessions over a 5-year period. Mrs. Kalish was alternately relieved and jealous of her husband's psychotherapeutic relationship. She wondered what *really* went on in those sessions. Soon after therapy ended, overt marital discord erupted and the couple divorced.

Depression is the most common psychiatric disorder seen in medical practice. Epidemiologic studies have shown that 5–15% of all patients who visit their family physician suffer from a major depression (21, 22). Depressed patients present with worrisome physical symptoms such as anorexia, fatigue, and weight loss. Depression may not be considered until after an occult malignancy work-up is completed. Depression can be difficult to diagnose, and despite the development of the DST, there is no reliable laboratory test to confirm the diagnosis in an outpatient setting (23).

Currently, a dominant explanation for depression is the biomedical model. According to this approach, depression is caused by an inheritable disorder of the regulation in neurotransmitters (primarily norepinephrine and serotonin) in the brain. The psychologic and social context of the patient is seen primarily as resulting from this disturbed metabolic state. The treatment is viewed by many physicians as being relatively simple and effective: medication that corrects these imbalances (tricyclic antidepressants and monoamine oxidase inhibitors). This model has great appeal to physicians who are trained in the biomedical model. They believe depression has become a medical disease that can be treated by a drug alone, without spending the time and effort to understand the precipitants of the illness or the patient's present life circumstances and social interactions.

Because of its simplicity and its organic focus, the biomedical model of depression has largely replaced its predecessor, the psychodynamic model, as the predominant approach to depression in primary care. The psychodynamic model views depression as arising from intrapsychic conflicts due to early childhood experiences. Treatment is focused on the past and attempts are made to resolve these conflicts by gaining insight into their origins. Unfortunately, this approach takes years of individual psychotherapy and is not readily amenable to use in primary care. Physicians who refer depressed patients for individual psychotherapy are rarely involved in the treatment process and may not receive follow-up on the patients.

Both of these approaches have contributed a great deal to our understanding of depression, but neither should be used in isolation. To view depression as merely a biochemical disturbance treatable by drugs alone is inadequate, yet many physicians treat depression without an understanding of the patient's life circumstances. A systems approach incorporates the biomedical and individual approaches, but also includes the family and larger social systems. It does not try to determine whether psychosocial factors are the result or the cause of the depression, but examines the interaction between the patient's symptoms and behaviors and his/her social context.

A Systems Approach to Depression

Rather than treating this patient only individually, Dr. E spoke to Mr. Kalish first and then asked to see his wife. Because she was sitting in the waiting room, Dr. E was able to spend the last half of the interview speaking to both Mr. and Mrs. Kalish. He learned from Mrs. Kalish that she was very worried about her usually active husband's recent spiral downward. She said he was a creature of habit but now seemed not to care about his usual routines or hobbies. Instead, he seemed preoccupied about a bad investment in the stock market and his perception that parents and school administrators did not appreciate his work. Mr. Kalish verified his wife's description, but said she should think less about him and get on with leading her own life.

When Dr. E asked what each member of this couple was doing to solve Mr. Kalish's problem, Mr. Kalish sat mute while Mrs. Kalish enthusiastically described the programs she had constructed to return her husband to his old self. These included an exercise program (Mrs. Kalish was an avid exerciser), a vitamin program (Mrs. Kalish herself sold vitamins), talking to her husband's colleagues to get them to encourage him, and generally being cheerful and supportive of her husband regardless of how she really felt. Mr. Kalish acknowledged he was unresponsive to all these efforts. In fact, it seemed the more she tried to cheer him up the more depressed he became. As Dr. E saw this familiar pattern unfold, he recognized that Mr. Kalish was feeling quite inadequate—and quite angry—at work, at home, and generally with himself. He felt his wife did not understand, that she, like others, did not see behind his facade, that she did not realize how inadequate he truly was underneath. The couple's life had developed into a well-meaning, but vicious cycle of the husband feeling badly and complaining, the wife trying to cheer him up and invalidating his feelings in the process, the husband feeling angry and withdrawing, and the cycle repeating itself.

Given Mr. Kalish's vegetative signs, and the individual and family dynamics of this case, Dr. E decided on the following treatment plan. First, he referred Mr. and Mrs. Kalish to a psychotherapist who would see Mr. Kalish individually as well as seeing Mr. and Mrs. Kalish as a couple. Dr. E explained to the couple that Mrs. Kalish could help with her husband's treatment. From past experience, Dr. E was familiar with the work of this psychotherapist and agreed to attend the first session with this couple to help the referral along, provide information, and demonstrate that he and the therapist were working together to treat Mr. Kalish. Second, Dr. E began Mr. Kalish on a low dose of antidepressants.

In the early months of treatment, Mrs. Kalish was enthusiastic and optimistic, as was her nature, about the psychotherapy. Mr. Kalish, on the other hand, was pessimistic and somewhat suspicious. Over time, in both the individual and conjoint sessions, Mr. Kalish learned that the therapist was able to listen to his despair and empathize without needing to cheer him up. In fact, the therapist encouraged him to focus on his depressed feelings and examine them closely during therapy so he could better relax outside of the sessions. With Mrs. Kalish, the therapist quickly discovered, as with most family members, that she had her own treatment plan for her husband—the "cheer-him-up" approach to depression. As often happens with this approach, Mrs. Kalish's treatment resulted in a worsening of the patient's symptoms. He felt she did not understand, isolating him further. (This same cycle can be set up between depressed patients and well-meaning physicians.) The therapist discussed what the couple termed their "communication problems" and prescribed nightly 10-minute sessions in which Mr. Kalish discussed any subject he wished and Mrs. Kalish listened, speaking only at the end to summarize what her husband had said and let him know she understood. Mrs. Kalish was delighted to play a role in her husband's treatment; Mr. Kalish was relieved that his wife was beginning to understand.

Treatment lasted 6 months and Mr. Kalish was successfully withdrawn from the antidepressant medication. He started his own exercise program with some buddies from work. His marriage improved along with his feelings about himself as a person. The use of both individual and conjoint psychotherapy, and the collaboration between the therapist and the physician, allowed for the most effective and efficient treatment of Mr. Kalish's depression.

A systems approach to problems such as depression does not stop at the organic or individual levels of the system, but views the problem as an important interpersonal event. In this case, Mr. and Mrs. Kalish were locked into a repetitive cycle in which Mrs. Kalish's "treatment" contributed to maintaining the problem. Watzlawick et al. theorized that most lingering behavioral problems begin inadvertently, then persist because people's solutions make the problem worse (24). Believing that the solution is not powerful enough, they do "more of the same," unintentionally perpetuating the problem. In this case, Mrs. Kalish began trying to help her husband first by being cheerful and encouraging. When that did not help, she escalated ("more of the same") by suggesting exercise and vitamins, and mobilizing his friends to also cheer him up. The more Mrs. Kalish did this, the more Mr. Kalish felt misunderstood, furthering his depression. It would have been easy for Dr. E to also respond to Mr. Kalish with a "cheerful" treatment strategy. However, by assessing that Mr. Kalish's solution was to try to avoid his depression and that Mrs. Kalish's solution was to cheer her husband up, Dr. E was able to formulate a workable treatment strategy using the patient and his family and involving a referral to a systems-oriented psychotherapist.

Alcoholism

A Biomedical Approach to Alcoholism

Mrs. Jones, a 55-year-old housewife and mother of 6 children, was admitted to the hospital for an elective cholecystectomy. The surgery was uneventful, but on her third postoperative day, she developed tachycardia and a fever of 102. She became confused and agitated, and had to be restrained in bed. Medical evaluation revealed no signs of infection or blood loss. The following day she began shouting about spiders on the wall of her room and refused to let her surgeon examine her. A psychiatrist was consulted and diagnosed delirium tremens (DTs). She was treated with large doses of haloperidol, a major tranquilizer, and gradually improved over the next 3 days. Her husband, an orthopedic surgeon at the hospital, revealed that his wife drank 3 to 4 drinks each night, but that she was never intoxicated and never drank early in the day. Her lab tests showed that she had a macrocytic anemia (folate and B_{12} levels had been ordered) and abnormal liver function tests, which had been attributed to her gallbladder disease. After her symptoms cleared,

Mrs. Jones was seen again by the psychiatrist, and the hospital's alcoholism counselor. While she admitted drinking "a couple of drinks" each night, she denied that she had a drinking problem, and complained to her surgeon and the director of the hospital when the psychiatrist suggested that she was alcoholic. She refused any treatment or follow-up for her drinking, but her husband agreed to monitor her drinking very closely for the next few months.

This case represents a common presentation of alcoholism in medical practice. Studies have shown that between 20% and 30% of all hospitalized patients suffer from alcoholism (25, 26), and that the disease has a major effect on health. Yet, alcoholism is rarely screened for, and classic syndromes such as DTs are often missed. For example, chronic alcohol ingestion causes an increase in the mean corpuscular volume of red blood cells, and studies have documented that alcoholism is a much more common cause of macrocytosis than are nutritional deficiencies (27). Yet physicians commonly order B_{12} and folate levels without asking the patient about his/her drinking.

The lack of awareness of alcoholism by health care providers is only part of the massive denial associated with the illness. As in this case, the patient usually denies he/she has a problem with drinking, drastically underreports alcohol consumption, and insists that he/she can stop drinking at any time. The patient will often flee from the physician who insists that he/she is an alcoholic, and find a physician who will ignore the problem, one who may be a heavy drinker as well. Families often share in the denial of the problem, ignoring or covering up the signs of alcohol abuse. The more family members who drink heavily, the more difficult treatment will be.

The disease concept of alcoholism has become increasingly popular in medicine, with mixed results. Alcoholism is described as a disorder, often inherited, in which the patient loses the ability to control his/her drinking. The patient is not held responsible for the drinking, but is encouraged to admit that he/she is powerless to change it and must accept the help of others. While this approach has allowed many patients to accept the diagnosis of alcoholism with less guilt, it has solidified the biomedical approach of physicians to alcoholism. Detailed psychosocial histories are rarely obtained. After the diagnosis is made, emphasis is placed upon confronting the alcoholic and forcing him/her into treatment. If this initial confrontation fails, the care provider may feel hopeless and give up on the patient, believing that he/she will not change. An effective approach to alcoholism requires an understanding of the context of the drinking: How does it affect the patient and other family members? What role does intoxicated behavior play in the family? Who else in the family drinks?

A Systems Approach to Alcoholism

During the hospitalization, Mrs. Jones' family physician, Dr. F, expressed his concern about her overall health to her husband. He urged Dr. Jones to ask all the important family members and friends to come to a meeting in the hospital to discuss Mrs. Jones' health. Dr. Jones first said he himself would relay any important information and that such a meeting was unnecessary. However, he agreed to invite these people when the family physician told both him and his wife that such a meeting often helped patients to implement a treatment plan and even prevent future hospitalizations.

The next evening the meeting took place. Attending were Dr. F, Dr. Jones, Mrs. Jones, the Jones' eldest married daughter, their two sons who were still living at home, Mrs. Jones' mother, who lived in the next town, her next-door neighbor, who was a close friend, and the hospital's alcoholism counselor. When everyone convened, Dr. F said Mrs. Jones had been quite ill and he was concerned that she have a good rehabilitation. Mrs. Jones' daughter asked what was wrong with her mother. Dr. F said, as he had previously told Dr. and Mrs. Jones, that Mrs. Jones lab tests were consistent with those found in people who were chronically drinking too much alcohol. He turned to Mrs. Jones and acknowledged she had denied having a drinking problem and said he was perplexed about her lab tests and concerned about how to prevent recurrences of her illness. Mrs. Jones' two sons immediately spoke up, saying they worried that both their parents drank too much. Slowly over the 30-minute meeting, each family member expressed their concern about Mrs. Jones' alcohol abuse. Dr. F continually spoke of the resources and strengths in this family. Toward the end, Mrs. Jones broke into tears and told of her own worries about herself and her husband.

A plan emerged at the end of the meeting for the same group to meet with a family therapist who had a special interest in alcohol problems. There was some resistance to this idea until Dr. F said he would attend the first meeting with them as the primary care doctor who had known them all for many years. The Jones' teenage sons expressed interest in going to an Al-Anon meeting, so Dr. F gave them information about a nearby group. The neighbor friend had herself been to an AA meeting with her cousin the previous year and suggested she go with Dr. and Mrs. Jones. Mrs. Jones agreed, though Dr. Jones refused, continuing to label his drinking as "social drinking." Anyway, he said he certainly could not afford to show his face at an AA meeting "for professional reasons."

The hospital meeting was the beginning of a slow recovery for this family. Mrs. Jones had several relapses, but eventually dealt with her alcohol problem. Dr. Jones continued to deny his problem until sometime after his wife successfully recovered and he had a heart attack. Again, the family met in the hospital and worked together to help him conquer his alcohol dependence as part of his cardiac rehabilitation.

In recent years, even the more traditional alcohol counselors have moved toward utilizing family systems as resources in dealing with alcoholic behavior. The confrontation of family and friends of Betty Ford is a classic example of the usefulness of activating relevant others as part of treatment. Rather than viewing the family interactions as either the cause (e.g., "she drove him to drink") or the result of alcoholism, systems theory considers chemical dependencies as symptoms of a dysfunctional family. Alcoholism plays an important stabilizing role in these families, and the families help to maintain (or "enable") the alcoholic behavior.

In a series of studies, Steinglass and his colleagues have studied alcoholism in families from a systems perspective. They hospitalized alcoholics and their spouses for 10 days on a special ward designed to be as much like home as possible with alcohol freely available (28). Each couple had recognizable patterns of interaction during sober and intoxicated states and predictably cycled from one to the other. During intoxication, the couple had a much greater range of affective communication. Drinking clearly had an adaptive function for these families (29). Berenson discussed the differences between "dry" (unemotional, boring) and "wet" (overexperiencing and irrational) states and the importance of integrating the two states for the individual and the family if the alcoholic is to recover permanently (30). In one study the amount of alcohol consumed correlated with marital satisfaction for steady drinkers (31).

Steinglass has developed a "life history model" of alcoholic families that describes different stages that these families pass through (32). In a naturalistic study, he periodically observed alcoholic families in their own homes over a 6-month period. He found that different patterns of family interactions were associated with different stages of alcoholism (33). Families in which the alcoholic drank throughout the 6 months of the study ("stable wet") were more disengaged and interacted very little and in a rigid fashion. Families in which the alcoholic was abstinent ("stable dry") exhibited midrange cohesion and the most flexible patterns of interaction. Families in which the alcoholic switched from drinking to abstinence or vice versa ("transitional") appeared enmeshed, with the greatest physical closeness and the narrowest range of content in their communications.

The family physician has the opportunity to make the early diagnosis of alcoholism, before the chronic social and medical complications occur. Baird has observed that the first sign of alcoholism is often family conflict, and that, in his practice, 80% of families with alcoholism had major conflicts (8). Baird suggested five steps for involving the family in the diagnosis and treatment of alcoholism (34):

1. *Be open to the diagnosis of alcoholism.* Up to 10% of the general population suffers from the disorder. Assessing the social context of medical problems assists in making the diagnosis.
2. *Take a family history.* Alcoholism runs in families and obtaining a genogram will establish the family context for the problem.
3. *Assemble the family.* During a hospitalization, the physician is in a particularly powerful position, and family meetings are most successful in this setting.
4. *Interview the family.* Whenever possible, let the family bring up the drinking problem, but avoid attempts at quantifying alcohol consumption. Focus on the family consequences of the drinking, and try to come to an agreement as to how much of a problem it is for the family. Offer direct referral to treatment facilities or information on community resources.
5. *Be honest about the diagnosis* by recording it in the patient's chart, and accept the limitations of medical practice, recognizing that alco-

holism is a chronic illness that takes years to develop and often years to treat.

For families like the Joneses, alcoholism can be an insidious and deadly disorder. The physician needs to be able to approach the individual, the family systems, and the treatment system with an understanding of the interactional dynamics that can underpin this problem and some knowledge of how to draw on the strengths of the systems to begin the process toward successful treatment.

Conclusions

We have presented these six examples to illustrate the processes and the approaches that can be used in applying systems theory to medicine. Some commonalities exist across these different examples in the ways the systems-oriented practitioners chose to define the problems as well as the methods they used for treatment.

First, the family is seen as both an important source of information and an important source of resources and strengths on which to draw during treatment. The biopsychosocial approach to diagnosis includes an analysis of both family life cycle issues confronting a symptomatic patient and the more acute stressors experienced by the family. Illness is viewed as always having a psychosomatic component. For this reason, all interviews should include a mix of biomedical and psychosocial questions to avoid somatic fixation by the physician or the patient or family. The biopsychosocial model recognizes that symptoms can be interpersonal events or communications. As in the depression example, the solution applied to these symptoms can inadvertently maintain the problem. What begins as a healthy response to an acute event can in the long term become unhealthy, as in the chronic illness example. The meaning given to the illness by the patient and the family and the role of the illness behavior are important parts of the practitioner's diagnostic work-up.

In addition to information gathering and assessment, the family or relevant system provides resources for managing compliance problems, such as in the diabetes example. Family members can help to implement (or block) needed life-style changes, such as in the cardiovascular disease and alcoholism examples.

Finally, understanding interpersonal dynamics and the interplay between different levels of systems can help the physician to maintain his/her own stability in the whirlwind of emotions that can accompany the diagnosis and treatment of illness and disease. The systems-oriented physician forms alliances with the patient *and* the family members. He/she typically does not keep secrets. The systems-oriented physician learns to recognize power struggles early and know that one can only change one's own behavior in the end. Also, with a pressured or mysterious case, the systems-oriented physician knows that collaboration offers both support and a new perspective on persistent symptoms.

References

1. Engel BL: The clinical application of the biopsychosocial model. Am J Psychiatry 1980;137:535–544.
2. Minuchin S, Baker L, Rossman BL, et al: A conceptual model of psychosomatic illness in children: Family organization and family therapy. Arch Gen Psychiatry 1975;32:1031–1038.
3. Minuchin S, Rosman BL, Baker L: Psychosomatic Families. Cambridge, MA, Harvard University Press, 1978, pp 21–50.
4. Baker L, Minuchin S, Rosman B: The use of beta adrenergic blockade in the treatment of psychosomatic aspects of juvenile diabetes mellitus, in Snart A (ed); Advances in Beta Adrenergic Blockade Therapy. Princeton, NJ, Excerpta Medica, 1974, pp 67–80.
5. Baker L, Minuchin S, Milman L, et al: Psychosomatic aspects of juvenile diabetes mellitus: A progress report. Mod Prob Paediatr 1975;12:332–343.
6. White K, Kolman ML, Wexler P, et al: Unstable diabetes and unstable families: A psychosocial evaluation of diabetic children with recurrent ketoacidosis. Pediatrics 1984;73:749–755.
7. Cerretto MC, Travis LB: Implications of psychological and family factors in the treatment of diabetes. Pediatr Clin North Am 1984;31:689–710.
8. Doherty WJ, Baird MA: Family Therapy and Family Medicine. New York, Guilford Press, 1983.
9. Morisky DE, Levine DM, Green LW, et al: Five year blood pressure control and mortality following health education for hypertensive patients. Am J Pub Health 1983;73:153–162.
10. Hoebel FC: Brief family interactional therapy in the management of cardiac related high risk behaviors. J Fam Pract 1976;3:613–618.
11. Medalie JH, Snyder M, Groen JJ, et al: Angina pectoris among 10,000 men: 5 year incidence and univariate analysis. Am J Med 1973;55:583–594.
12. Medalie JH, Goldbourt U: Angina pectoris among 10,000 men: Psychosocial and other risk factors as evidenced by a multivariate analysis of a five year incidence study. Am J Med 1976;60:910–921.
13. Patterson J: Critical factors affecting family compliance with home treatment for children with cystic fibrosis. Fam Relat 1985;34:78–90.
14. Heinzelman F, Bagley RW: Response to physical activity programs and their effects on health behavior. Pub Health Rep 1970;85:905–911.
15. Oakes TW, Ward JR, Gray RM, et al: Family expectation and arthritis patient compliance to a hand resting splint regimen. J Chron Dis 1970;22:757–764.
16. Doherty WJ, Schrott HG, Metcalf L, Iasiello Vailas L: Effect of spouse support and health beliefs on medication adherence. J Fam Pract 1983;17:837–841.
17. Doherty WJ, Baird MA: A protocol for family compliance counseling. Fam Syst Med 1984;2(3):333–336.
18. Penn P: Coalitions and binding interactions in families with chronic illness. Fam Syst Med 1983;1:16–25.
19. Sheinberg M: The family and chronic illness: A treatment diary. Fam Syst Med 1983;1(2):26–36.

20. Van Eijk J, Grol R, Huygen F, et al: The family doctor and the prevention of somatic fixation. Fam Syst Med 1983;1(2):5–15.
21. Reifler BV, Okimoto JT, Heidrich FE, Invi TS: Recognition of depression in a university based family medicine residency program. J Fam Pract 1979;9:623–628.
22. Hoeper EW, Nycz GR, Cleavy PD, et al: Estimated prevalence of RDC mental disorders in primary medical care. Int J Ment Health 1978;8(2):6–15.
23. Hirschfeld RMA, Koslow SH, Kupfer DJ: The clinical utility of the dexamethosone suppression test in psychiatry. Summary of a National Institute of Mental Health workshop. JAMA 1983;250:2172–2174.
24. Watzlawick P, Weakland JH, Fisch R: Change: Principles of Problem Formation and Problem Resolution. New York, Norton, 1974.
25. Tennant FS, Day CM, Ungerleider JT: Screening for drug and alcohol abuse in a general medical population. JAMA 1979;242:533.
26. Sherin KM, Piotrowski MS, Panek SM, Doot MC: Screening for alcoholism in a community hospital. J Fam Pract 1982;15:1091–1095.
27. Chick J, Kreitman N, Plant M: Mean cell volume and gamma glutamyl transpeptidase as markers of drinking in working men. Lancet 1981;1:1249–1951.
28. Steinglass P, Davis D, Berenson D: Observations of conjointly hospitalized alcoholic couples during sobriety and intoxication: Implications for theory and practice. Fam Process 1977;16:1–16.
29. Davis D, Berenson D, Steinglass P, Davis S: The adaptive consequences of drinking. Psychiatry 1974;37:209–215.
30. Berenson D: Alcohol and the family system, in Guerin P (ed): Family Therapy: Theory and Practice. New York, Gardner Press, 1976 pp 284–297.
31. Jacob T, Dunn NJ, Leonard K: Patterns of alcohol abuse and family stability. Alcoholism: Clin Exp Res 1983;7:382–385.
32. Steinglass PA: A life history model of the alcoholic family. Fam Process 1980;19:211–226.
33. Steinglass P: The alcoholic family at home: Patterns of interaction of dry, wet, and transitional stages of alcoholism. Arch Gen Psychiatry 1981;138:578–584.
34. Baird MA: Chemical dependency: A protocol for involving the family. Fam Syst Med 1985;3(2):216–220.

CHAPTER 7

Systems-oriented Counseling

Karen Weihs and Karen Kingsolver

When a factory worker complains to his/her family physician of a sore throat, back pain, and irritability at home, the physician can choose to work up the sore throat and the back pain, using a straightforward biomedical approach. Alternatively, in addition to biomedical problems, the clinician can consider broader diagnoses such as job stress, marital discord, and depression. When a patient with well-controlled chronic heart failure presents with trouble sleeping and crying spells, without dyspnea, ankle edema, or chest pain, the physician can reassure the patient that his/her chronic disease is under control and leave it at that, or he/she can address the way these symptoms are part of more generalized distress in the patient's life.

The primary care physician assesses many patients with multiple, often vague complaints. Symptoms ranging from pains in the feet to a child's reluctance to go to school are part of everyday practice. The biomedical model allows the physician to diagnose specific well-defined medical conditions and to rule out others, but many symptoms will be left unaddressed if the biomedical model is the only one used to take care of patients.

In this chapter we will describe a model that allows physicians to understand and work with all of the symptoms presented by their patients. The systems model focuses on the complex human interactions that intertwine with each medical problem (1). Through exploring the broader context of illness, the physician can compose an integrated picture of a patient's situation and plan solutions that fit the patient's real life experience.

The Symptom Reflects the System

How does the patient experience his/her illness? An individual's experience of health and illness is formed by his/her own responses to his/her problems, and by the responses of family and friends. People respond naturally to changes within their bodies and to changes in their environment. As a patient describes a symptom, he/she recalls his/her physical sensations, emotions and behavior around the symptom, and thoughts about the meaning of the symptom. He/she can also recall the reactions of family members and friends, and may or may not be aware of how they shaped the way he/she coped with the symptom.

Because the family is the primary emotional system for most people, understanding human experience requires understanding the family. Through their interactions with the patient during an illness, family members act out characteristic patterns based on past experiences in the family. The physician who explores these responses to the patient's symptoms will, therefore, encounter a sample of family life that represents their unique way of relating to illness.

Physicians often cut the patient short before he/she gets to the part of his/her story that includes the family reactions, and they seldom inquire about family responses if the patient does not volunteer them (2,3). Even experienced clinicians who are aware of the importance of family factors tend to overfocus on the patient's perceptions of the family, and often neglect to find out about the thoughts, feelings, and behavior of other family members.

Clinical Example #1: Child with Febrile Seizures

The family systems medicine model is illustrated by a family physician's approach to a 14-month-old child who had recurrent seizures brought on by high fevers. The child received a medical work-up to evaluate neurologic abnormalities, and the physician recommended treatment with phenobarbital to prevent further seizures. When family members were asked about their reaction to the seizures, it became obvious that the parents, grandparents, aunts, uncles, and neighbors were all very concerned about the child. Furthermore, they needed a way of understanding the situation so that they knew how to treat him.

The physician surmised that how she discussed the child's problem with them might strongly influence whether the child was parented in a health-promoting or an illness-inducing way. She couched the problem as a temporary difficulty for a basically healthy child, instead of as an enduring handicap for a vulnerable child in need of constant protection. The physician had observed the parents' responses to their child, to each other, to the relatives, and to the physician herself, and anticipated the challenges they faced in changing their thinking, feelings, and behaviors toward their child. Because she was aware of specific ways in which the child might be overprotected, the physician asked the parents to plan particular healthy interactions with the child.

If the family doctor had ignored the family system, the child may have been overprotected for no valid medical reason. Years later the physician may have then been faced with a child who developed stomach pains whenever he was sent to kindergarten, and who was frightened to be without his mother. His mother, thinking of and treating her child as sickly, may have been anxious whenever he was out of her sight, and she may have insisted that the doctor conduct an elaborate medical investigation of the new problem.

At the latter stage, overinvolvement of mother and child would be much harder for them to change. Tremendous time and effort would be required for the child to develop more adaptive interactions with his family, teachers, and peers. By understanding the family and the possible consequences of a new problem in the child, the physician addresses the total treatment needs in the family, which helps family members develop in a healthy way.

By exploring the symptom within its unique context, the physician sometimes gets the chance to foster lasting changes in patients' health. In this chapter, we will refer to this process of exploring for opportunities and mining the discovered pay dirt as counseling. Counseling is an interaction between a clinician and someone seeking help for a problem, with the mutual goal of solving the problem.

Systems-oriented counseling is based on understanding how individuals exist and evolve within their own unique biomedical, familial, and psychosocial settings. Systems-oriented counseling uses the context of the problem and the details of the relationships between physician, patient, family, and community to understand the problem and formulate solutions.

Clinical Example #2: Daughter with Stomach Pain, Mother with Cancer

The following family physician encounter illustrates how a patient's family system impacts on her experience of her own health. The physician unobtrusively helps the patient tell her story.

In the physician's initial visit with Sue, a 35-year-old single parent with two children, a 10-year-old daughter Amy, and a 7-year-old son Chad, Dr. W began the interview by chatting with the patient about where she lived and about her experience in getting to the office. She then asked the reason for the patient's visit. The interview then proceeded as below:

PT: Well, I haven't had a checkup for three years and I would like to find out if the pain in my stomach is anything to worry about.

DR: Tell me more about your concerns.

PT: Well, I've generally been a healthy person, and I eat well. I get some exercise at the health spa at least twice a week, and I've only been hospitalized twice in my life when my children were born.

DR: It sounds like you're taking good care of yourself and that includes coming in for a checkup.

PT: Well, I really don't want to end up like my mother when I'm fifty-five, so I thought I'd better come in.

DR: Your mother?

PT: Yes, she just found out that she has breast cancer and is having radiation treatments starting next week. She had a terrible time after the mastectomy, with an infection in the wound, and she got so depressed.

DR: Sounds like you've been through a lot lately.

PT: Yes, I guess I have. I hadn't really thought about it. I'm pretty close to my mom and I hate to see her suffer. I think she's through the tough part now, so I can start thinking about my own life again.

DR: You've been so worried about her that you haven't noticed what a strain you've been under.

PT: Um-hm. The kids have been a big help to me. They never used to clean up after dinner or do their homework without being told. Now they're doing those things regularly. It seems like they knew that I really needed the help and were able to come through.

DR: You're obviously a sensitive family. You noticed your mom's distress over her cancer treatment and felt sad that she was having such a hard time. Your kids seem to have noticed that you needed some extra help and did their best to make life easier for you.

PT: Yeah, we do stick together. I'm pretty lucky.

DR: You certainly are.

In the interaction above, the physician–patient system operates smoothly so that the patient's presenting problem unfolds in its life context. By actively listening the physician gleaned a wealth of information about the patient's life in a short time. In only 2 minutes the physician learned that Sue has been coping with changes in her family system related to her mother's cancer. Though she presented her stomach pain as the problem, she quickly mentioned significant events of her recent life.

In a family systems approach, all parts of the patient's presentation are considered meaningful for healing. The mutual influencing of symptoms of illness, stress, and family function are evident in Sue's description of the situation. At this stage a sorting process begins, in which the physician and patient work together to discover how the bits of information fit together to explain the problem.

Knowing that any kind of pain can be brought on or made worse by stress, the physician might guess that the stress of Sue's mother's recent cancer diagnosis and treatment has upset the way the family functions, and is related to the stomach pain. At this point in the interview, it is unclear what changes have occurred and how they are stressful for the patient. Hypotheses can be generated about the interactions of the patient, her children, her mother, and the family physician. These hypotheses would address the impact of changes in the patient's health as they affect and are affected by other members of the system.

It could be that she is worried that she, too, will develop cancer. She may be physically fatigued from the increased time demands (on top of the many stresses of being a single parent), and unable to find a way to get enough rest. The anxiety over the possible death of her mother may be preventing her from relaxing, even though she has the time for it. The change in her children's behavior may be accompanied by a feeling of distance from them if taking care of them was her only way of being close.

With these hypotheses in mind, the physician can continue the interview with a problem-oriented biomedical review, together with a focus on the family response to the patient. While proceeding, the clinician remains open to new information that would confirm, modify, or refute the tentative hypotheses, or that would suggest entirely new hypotheses. The remainder of the chapter will describe the thinking and behavior of the physician doing systems-oriented counseling in primary care.

The thinking process used for understanding the problem begins at the first contact of the physician with the patient. We will therefore begin with a way to identify the levels of the system that have been changed with a particular problem. We will then focus on the characteristics of systems that are useful in assessing changes at the family and wider social levels.

The behavioral skills for involving the patient, exploring the problem, and designing a plan will then be outlined. First we describe essential skills for all physicians, including referral of patients whose problems require family level change that cannot be made with a straightforward educational intervention. We then discuss more advanced skills that can be acquired by those who want to deal more extensively with family problems.

The position of the physician in the patient's life is the subject of the last section of the chapter. Levels of responsibility for the physician and the patient will be related to the type of problem being worked on. Methods will be suggested for the physician to monitor his/her own impact on the patient and on the patient's family system.

Primary Care Contexts and the Need for Family Involvement

Primary care practice involves five types of patient visits:

- well child
- adult health maintenance
- prenatal
- acute illness, complaint, or problem
- chronic illness, complaint, or problem

The primary care physician who uses a systems approach guides his/her depth of exploration and involvement in family issues to some extent by the type of visit. For a given visit, the key to an appropriate discussion of family matters is a quick assessment of the current amount of change in the family, and of the amount of strain associated with the stressful changes. The stress of change can foster growth and creativity if the person and his/her family have the needed physical, emotional, intellectual, and behavioral resources to adapt to the new situation in positive ways.

On the other hand, the need for change can bring distress and system breakdown if important coping resources are lacking. Failure to change and grow can have serious consequences, including illness. The appropriate type and amount of intervention in the family system is that which allows the family to continue to function and grow in the face of the change required to solve the presenting problem.

During well child, health maintenance, and prenatal visits, the physician can profitably review the predicted developmental changes in the family and discuss the family's resources for coping with them. Visits for acute and chronic illness vary widely in the extent and type of family involvement needed to solve the problems at hand. A symptom of illness can stem from an outside stressor, or it can indicate distress within the family system. If the family is unable to cope with an outside stressor, other symptoms may arise as the family system moves from a functional equilibrium or homeostasis to a disequilibrium or dysfunctional equilibrium.

A symptom may also indicate preexisting dysfunction in the family itself. In this case, the symptom is thought to indicate that some change or anticipated change in the family threatens to upset its equilibrium. The anxiety about this change activates conflicts within the family that cannot be resolved, and are therefore expressed as symptoms. Symptoms can be either a means of preventing a threatened change, or a way for a change to take place (4).

One role of the physician is to help the family anticipate problems in coping and plan for bringing in new resources to prevent family dysfunction if necessary. When family dysfunction already exists, an appropriate role for the physician is to identify the problem at the family level and work with the patient and family to restore healthy family function, to the extent this is feasible. This can be done in a family counseling session conducted by the family physician or by referring the family to a family therapist.

Anticipatory Guidance for Developmental Changes

Developmental changes are predictable. Families attempt to adjust to meet the different needs of each new stage of the life cycle. Many resources are available to guide the family physician in anticipating normal stages of individual and family development (5). Although generalizations are useful for thinking about possibilities and opening discussion with patients, each situation is unique. From family to family there is wide variation in the amount of stress caused by particular life changes, and in the usefulness of specific coping strategies for the family. While it is often therapeutic to tell the patient and the family that stress and change are normal and that other people struggle with similar issues, such reassurance can be most effective after the clinician fully understands the patient's own situation, with its special flavor and dilemmas.

Coping with Health Problems as Additional Stressors

Some biomedical problems affect the family system as new stresses. If the family of a 12-year-old boy who breaks his arm playing basketball has adequate resources to cope with this episode, it will provide the care he needs during his recovery. With many families, the physician may need to inquire only briefly into family functioning to establish its adequacy to deal with the situation smoothly. In this type of medical encounter, as well as all other types, one of the roles of the family physician is to discuss the manner in which the family will provide for the new needs of the patient.

Comprehensive anticipatory guidance for medical stresses in a family system addresses both instrumental and emotional needs of the patient and the family. Instrumental needs include such activities as extra trips to the doctor's office and arrangement of new ways of performing regular duties (e.g., schoolwork) during the time of disability. Emotional needs include the desirability of family members coping positively with the emotional response to illness by the patient and other family members.

For many health problems managed by the primary care physician, discussing associated changes with the patient reveals that the family system has the ability to respond effectively to all the demands of the illness. Anticipating these changes allows the patient and the family to actively take charge, rather than being additionally stressed by surprising repercussions of the illness. Educating patients and families in a timely way about potential problems of coping can prevent many of these potential problems from becoming serious complications of the illness.

Inability to Cope with the Stress of Health Problems

In some cases the family is unable to cope satisfactorily with a new illness stressor. Difficulty in coping can be due to preexisting dysfunction of the family system, and inadequate coping can precipitate new family dysfunction. At times dysfunction manifests as symptoms in other family members. Huygen, a Dutch family physician, linked the clustering of doctor visits by multiple family members to stresses that exceeded the family's ability to cope (6).

It is not always possible to anticipate coping difficulties at the outset of illness. Checking on the family's coping at each visit and asking the patient to call in case of family distress can give the physician additional chances to detect coping difficulties and help families adjust better to illness.

The Problem as an Indicator of Family Dysfunction

When a symptom is thought to indicate dysfunction of the family system, systemic thinking is useful for understanding the connection between the two (7,8). All members of a family system influence, and are influenced by, one another, and by their own previous behavior, feelings, and thoughts. These interactions maintain the dynamic balance of life between changing and staying the same.

Some of the overall characteristics of every family are reflected in the personalities of individual family members. These persistent overall characteristics help the family maintain its identity. At the same time, the family constantly evolves as its members grow older. The dynamic equilibrium between changing and staying the same determines how well the family provides the flexibility to grow along with the stability to be secure.

As the balance in the family is upset by some change, a symptom may develop. A symptom often indicates that some change or anticipated change in the family is threatening to upset the equilibrium. The anxiety about this change activates conflicts that have been lying dormant. These conflicts, rather than being acknowledged and dealt with, are often expressed through symptoms. Patients who present symptoms to physicians are frequently unaware of the conflict and often oblivious to their family's avoidance of dealing with conflict. Symptoms are usually seen by patients as things separate from their personal relationships, foreign elements that can be banished irrespective of the family.

A family in which the oldest daughter is preparing to leave for college may be dysfunctional if the child has been the primary emotional support for her overtaxed mother. The mother may present to her physician with severe headaches that prevent her from doing her daily work. Through exploring the family's reaction to the headaches, the physician might discover that the headaches and resulting disability are threatening to block her daughter's leaving home. Uncovering the anxiety about the separation of mother and daughter (on everyone's part) gives them the chance to redefine their relationship, either on their own or in counseling.

The father and other children may be equally apprehensive about the departure of mother's main emotional support. The entire family, not just mother and daughter, could benefit from examining this issue prior to its contributing to serious problems for them. In this way the headache symptom can trigger the family system to change in ways that allow it to meet current and future family needs more satisfactorily (3). Recognizing family dysfunction in this case makes it possible for the family to solve a problem being expressed as a somatic symptom.

Because many patients do not appreciate the connections between symptoms and family matters, and do not volunteer this part of the history, it is necessary to systematically gather information about family members and significant others, especially as they interact with the patient around the symptom. This information will allow the physician to describe how the symptom helps keep the family stable, or helps the family change. The next step is to figure out how a change in the symptom (improvement or worsening) might affect the family system.

When the symptom is thought to reflect family dysfunction, the clinician needs to formulate a plan to investigate the family system. In many instances a family meeting is the best way to do this. If it is impossible to gather the family together because of death or distance, or if a family meeting would endanger the patient (such as in some cases of spouse or child abuse), the clinician can still work with the patient in the context of the family.

How much and in what way this kind of family counseling is done will depend on the time availability, interest, and skill of the physician. Family counseling may be done in small pieces over time as part of regular office visits, or it may involve more lengthy and intense special visits designed specifically to solve the problem by helping the patient understand and change his/her family interactions. Many physicians may wish to refer patients who need this kind of intensive family counseling. Specific referral skills will be discussed later in the chapter.

Using Systems Concepts with Symptoms Indicating Family Dysfunction

The long-term functioning of a family system depends on its ability to maintain itself and to provide for the needs of its individual members. The experience of each person and each family can be described in terms of their particular and collective ideas, feelings, and behaviors. The dominant experiences develop and maintain the family system, and are therefore the ones to explore during counseling efforts to solve a presenting problem.

Keeping in mind a framework of characteristics of family systems can help the physician listen for conflicts within the family. After a thorough systems-oriented interview, any family can be described in terms of key characteristics: wholeness, organization, patterning, and evolution. Each of these features will now be discussed, using the simplified system of an adult male and female in a newly forming couple relationship.

Wholeness

The new couple as a family system is more than a collection of individuals, and has an identity of its own. This characteristic of wholeness develops through the interchange of ideas, feelings, and behaviors between two people. A set of rules for this family system evolves from each person's family of origin, societal norms, and the couple's experience with one another. These rules usually arise without a conscious choice by the family members, and are very specific in determining how the system functions.

Because each person contributes components that are important to them, the new system is experienced as a blended whole, not necessarily a harmonious one, but a whole nonetheless. Tolerating differences and respecting each other's values, priorities, and feelings generate a sense of integrity, or consensual wholeness within the relationship. Some people appear to seek partners with very similar values, while others are attracted to persons with differing personal values about major life issues (e.g., sex, work, parenting, money).

Moderately divergent views of the world can actually complement each other and result in an overall balanced family stance. With one partner being more trusting, and one being more sceptical and cautious, the family can connect with the world optimistically, while being on guard against danger and exploitation. This is one of several characteristics for which people often marry somewhat opposite types from themselves. If one spouse regards the world with extreme distrust, while the other spouse considers the world to be basically benign, the stage is set for acute and chronic conflict over how to interact with others outside the home. When individuals do not respect and support each other's differences, the wholeness of the system is threatened.

The characteristic of wholeness is evaluated by trying to discern the rules for a couple's relationship. To figure out the unspoken rules that shape a couple's interactions, the clinician solicits each person's version of how men and women work out the instrumental and emotional logistics of living together (Who's the boss? How are decisions to be made? What are the life goals? Whose career is more important?)

In working with patients' symptoms in medical practice, physicians quickly realize that the rules pertaining to illness and health maintenance behavior vary greatly from family to family, and between individuals within families. Family members can work together in the healing process more effectively if they resolve intolerable differences and support each other's manner of becoming well and staying healthy. If all family members understand each others' health needs, the physician's efforts to maintain and improve everyone's health will pay off to a greater degree than if everyone tries to go it on their own.

Family members' ability to work together to make needed changes will determine how likely it is that any member's problems are solved. When listening to a patient describe a medical problem, the systems-oriented physician keeps in mind that all individual symptoms occur in a family system, and that the rules of the system as a whole, not just those of one or two members, determine the potential for growth and change.

Organization

The organization of a system is described by its structural elements, referred to as boundaries, subsystems, hierarchy, and alliances (9). These elements are related to two more global organizational properties—adaptability and cohesion.

The *boundary* of a family defines it as discrete from other systems, similar to the way city limits delineate municipalities. Interactions between subsystems within a system are governed by boundary rules. The amount of interchange across boundaries (permeability) is regulated to maintain a balance between the extremes of isolation and engulfment. For instance, a new couple may take advice and financial assistance from the wife's parents without difficulty when it is given freely, with respect for the couple, and when the couple can accept the help in a way that is comfortable for them. The boundary between these nuclear families is clear—well-defined, but allowing flexible interaction. By contrast, if the husband's parents try to impose help without regard for the couple's wants or needs, the couple may reject their attempts to help, generating anger and eventual withdrawal by those parents. In the latter situation, a more rigid boundary exists between the couple and the husband's parents, and their interactions will be less flexible.

Rigid boundaries may be workable for both sides if they keep their interactions fairly stereotypical and avoid conflict areas. The extended family system will be strained, however, if the parents are called on to help in a new way. Such a strain could arise if the husband's parents in the example above want their daughter-in-law to stay at home, and are asked instead to care for their grandchildren while the mother works. System strain may manifest as feelings of emotional and physical discomfort for one or several members of the family.

If the strain is too difficult to resolve unassisted, the problem may be brought to the doctor to be fixed. In the above situation, the grandmother may bring a 1-year-old grandchild to the doctor frequently for minor upper respiratory infections, rashes, and the like because of her own anxiety and ambivalence about being responsible for the child. The physician who understands the meaning of the symptom in the family system can facilitate the family's solving the problem.

An example of the opposite extreme would be a couple that chronically depended on one or both sets of parents for financial and emotional support. The insufficiently clear boundaries in such families are diffuse; there is too much interaction between the systems, and not enough autonomy within the system for the individuals or the family to conduct responsible and healthy lives. Most decisions are made by consulting with parents and other influential relatives and deferring to their opinions. Members of such families are also very prone to having symptoms when stress increases and an intolerable level of strain develops. They also do poorly when their sources of advice and support become ill or die.

Subsystems are membership groups within the larger system. In the preceding example, the generational boundary defines the parental and the new couple subsystems of the extended family system. Nuclear families contain several subsystems, including parental, marital, sibling, and parent–child. Subsystems are defined by shared characteristics of the members, as well as generalized differences from members of other subsystems. Individuals within subsystems have their own interpersonal boundaries, in addition to the boundary around the subsystem. As with systems, subsystems carry out their functions most effectively when their members have clear individual boundaries.

The *cohesion* of a system is characterized by how clear the boundaries are between one individual and another, as well as by the clarity of the boundaries between one subsystem and another. Healthy families have clear, flexible boundaries that evolve over time, adjusting appropriately to changes within and outside the family. For example, the healthy family gradually relaxes its hold on maturing adolescents, while maintaining clear rules regarding acceptable behavior while the teenager still resides with the family.

The extremes of cohesion are called *enmeshment* (very cohesive) and *disengagement* (not at all cohesive). *Enmeshed families* have a rigid boundary between the family and the outside world, and diffuse boundaries between family members. Sameness and agreement are valued above, and at the expense of, individuation. Members of enmeshed families are prone to respond to stress by somatizing, since they are overly attuned to changes in each other's sensations and emotions.

Disengaged families have diffuse boundaries between the family and the world, and rigid boundaries between individual family members. Disengaged families emphasize maintaining the appearance of emotional distance and separateness at the expense of healthy connectedness within a system or subsystem. The apparent emotional distance may actually reflect considerable underground emotional intensity, and may generate as much or more serious illness in the long run as do overt conflict and dependency. Members of disengaged families are particularly vulnerable to becoming depressed.

Hierarchy is a structural element defined by the amount of influence an individual or subsystem has on another individual or subsystem. The rules for establishing and maintaining hierarchy are generally based on family tradition and may be refractory to conscious intervention. For example, in a typical healthy family hierarchy, parents have greater influence than children.

Hierarchies are complex, however, and appearances are misleading. In

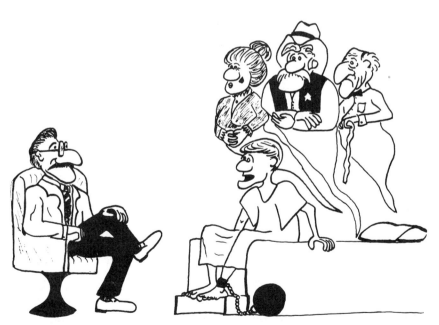

"My family? No problem. They go their way and I go mine."

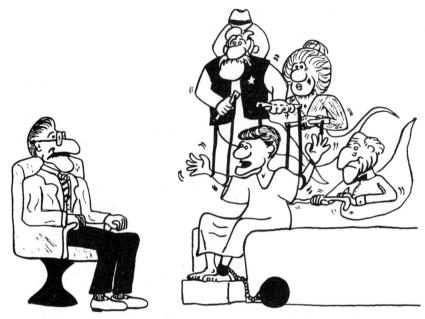

"My family? Oh, we're very close."

many families that are overtly father-dominated (patriarchal), mothers who are homemakers wield considerable power indirectly, through their "delegated" home domain and through their children. Part of the past male dominance had been economic—the "I'm the breadwinner, so I'm the boss" argument. The mass influx of women into the outside-the-home work force over the past three decades has shifted this part of traditional hierarchical relationships in ways that continue to evolve.

In the new couple system, the most functional hierarchical arrangement is complementary, where each partner has areas of expertise and greater influence that are welcomed and respected by the other. A complementary hierarchy shifts with the area of activity or issue, and it is generally clear who is in charge at a given time. In a symmetrical hierarchy the partners have similar strengths and weaknesses, and they compete for greater influence in both their strong and weak areas. This results in a less stable system, as the hierarchy shifts uncertainly from area to area and more doubt persists about who is in charge now and who will be in charge in the near future.

Alliances define the structure of a system through the closeness or distance between individuals and subsystems. Sharing ideas, feelings, and behaviors builds relationships experienced as alliances. Understanding shared as well as differentiating characteristics contributes both to a person's sense of individuality and to a sense of belonging to a group. The balance of difference versus sameness in individuals is different for every family. Changes in this balance occur throughout the life cycle.

The dynamic liveliness of the changing balance between conformity and individuality is referred to as the *adaptability* of the system. In a flexible system, the alliances serve the purpose of helping define the identity of family members, and the system allows for new alliances when appropriate. Daughters and mothers in flexible families with clear boundaries, for example, tend to become closer during early adolescence, while issues around puberty and sexuality make father–daughter interactions somewhat awkward. As peer interactions ascend in importance and conflict arises between the independence-seeking midadolescent and protective mother, the intensity of emotion may call for a decrease in time spent together by mother and daughter, or a change in the way time is spent together. Flexible families work these things out satisfactorily in the long run, though not without appreciable anguish at times.

A rigid family system includes alliances that do not evolve functionally over time. The lack of healthy evolution can contribute to the formation of symptoms in some family members. If a shift in alliances cannot be made, the resulting conflict and anxiety may manifest as physical symptoms (abdominal pain, headaches, chest pain, hyperventilation episodes, vasovagal syncope, etc.) Failure to modify alliances in a healthy way can generate dysfunctional family interactions also. In a rigid family the close father–daughter alliance typical of preadolescent girls may evolve to incest if the couple relationship is not meeting the needs of both spouses adequately.

When emotional tension increases between two people who are close, but who cannot resolve their differences, they commonly draw a third person into the emotional field. This process is called *triangulation*. For example, a young couple in their first year of marriage disagreed about how to spend their time on Saturday. The husband wanted to do the shopping and errands as a twosome. He saw the time as an opportunity to get reacquainted. Both people worked at very busy jobs during the week. The wife favored efficiency and thought they should go their own ways in order to accomplish more tasks. Her mother agreed with her and mother and daughter often talked about the daughter's inefficient husband. Saturday morning arguments included the issue of the husband's negative feelings about his mother-in-law. We will discuss how triangulation involves the physician later in the chapter.

The tension of a disagreement like the one above can be handled in many ways. Previous experiences with family and friends strongly influence how a couple deals with conflict. When unable to get his/her way unassisted, a person who is accustomed to winning without needing to compromise is likely to call in another person who agrees with him/her. The third person may offer moral support or even help argue that person's point of view against the partner. The dyadic relationship is weakened when one member allies with someone outside the dyad. Triangulation decreases the possibility of resolving a particular conflict within the dyad, and it reduces the chances that future conflicts will be dealt with effectively by the couple alone. The primary care physician frequently sees patients who could solve their problems more easily by disentangling their established dysfunctional triangles and avoiding forming new ones in future conflict situations.

Patterning

Patterning of a couple's behavior develops as each person finds ways to stimulate the other to produce the responses most desired. These patterns of behavior evolve over time, but the patterns that maintain the system and help it to evolve will tend to persist and become repetitive, even stereotyped. An outside observer can detect patterns of behavior that do not seem obvious to family members themselves. One typical pattern might describe how a couple decides what to do on the weekend. One partner brings the subject up for discussion and the other one offers several suggestions. The first partner chooses the two most desirable options, and the second partner makes the final decision. If this pattern of decision making results in satisfying experiences, it will be repeated and established as the dominant pattern for making decisions of this type.

Patterning also occurs in individuals' emotional experience. Feelings generated during initial interactions often resemble feelings of excitement and/or comfort experienced in each person's previous intimate relationships. The experience of being with this person in a new relationship becomes associated with familiar feelings, and a new self-reinforcing pattern has begun. These feeling patterns may actually be unpleasant in some respects, but sometimes their familiarity outweighs their negative aspects. A daughter of an alcoholic father, for example, will often establish intimate relationships with one or more men who are alcoholic, or who become alcoholic during the course of the relationship. In such instances, there are positive features, as well as negative characteristics of the relationships that are familiar to the woman. Some of the ways in which such a woman relates to her husband may actually facilitate the husband's being alcoholic, though the woman is unaware of her role in perpetuating the alcoholic family system. (See Chapter 6 for more about alcoholic families.)

Evolution

With the passage of time, every family encounters developmental changes and life stresses. In many cases the system is capable of adapting to these changes, with a variable amount of dis-ease. As mentioned above, this adaptation can be facilitated by anticipatory guidance from the physician. Change made by members of the system simply doing certain things differently is called first order change (5).

In some cases the system cannot accommodate to change adequately without changing itself so that its members can continue to flourish. At these times the system characteristics of wholeness, organization, and patterning evolve in ways called second order change. The necessary changes involve family members' *being* different, rather than just *doing* something differently (5). In the following hypothetical case, the family might adapt to new demands by making a first order change, or they might need to make a second order change at a deeper level.

A couple may experience difficulties in their sexual relationship after the man begins an antihypertensive medication that makes it more difficult for him to get and sustain an erection. One way to respond to the situation is for the man to describe his need for increased stimulation to his wife, who then may change her behavior in response. If the couple talks about their sexual experience and about what they need from each other, the new situation can be accommodated within the existing patterns of the system. The adjustments made by this couple are first order changes.

However, if strong feelings of embarassment inhibit both partners from verbalizing their needs, a change in the basic feeling and behavior patterns of the couple is needed to adapt to the situation. This second order change sometimes occurs spontaneously, but it requires more flexibility and resourcefulness than does first order change. When a family needs to make second order changes but cannot do so unassisted, an intervention by a person trained in family systems therapy is usually needed. The primary care physician can provide information for individuals to use in making first order changes, such as telling the patient that changes in sexual function may occur and helping him plan what to say to his wife. The physician may also facilitate first order change by meeting with the partners together to assure that they both understand the information and that their communication skills are adequate for planning and making changes.

Characteristics of a System

The following conceptual outline can be a valuable tool for gathering and recording information during a family systems–oriented counseling session. It can be used for understanding the problem and its possible solutions within the family ecology.

Wholeness
    Family ancestry—Record as genogram (see Chapter 8)
    Shared values and view of the world
Organization
    Boundaries ⎫ Contribute to cohesion, ranging from enmeshed to dis-
    Subsystems ⎭   engaged
    Hierarchy ⎫ Contribute to adaptability, ranging from rigid to flexible
    Alliances ⎭
Patterning—repetitive behavioral, ideational, and emotional sequences
Evolution
    First order change—occurs mostly within life cycle stages

Second order change—occurs mostly during transitions from one life cycle
stage to another, or with major changes in health status

Counseling for Problems Indicating Family Distress

The implicit contract between the physician and the patient is to prevent
predictable problems and to solve the problems that do occur. A problem-
oriented approach to counseling serves this purpose well. If the physician
in the opening scenario of the chapter considered the possibility of job
stress, marital discord, and depression in the factory worker with a sore
throat and irritability, she would need more skills than those used for a
strictly biomedical approach to the problem. To explore the patient's experience of illness in its family context, the physician gathers and integrates
information on three levels—behavioral, emotional, and ideational (what
people do, feel, and think). The physician's method of exploring the illness
with the patient will influence the solutions that are considered by patient
and physician. We will describe a systematic method of gathering information to build a broad base of understanding for working toward solutions.

The physician can develop counseling skills to any level on a continuum
of sophistication (10). Moving along the continuum involves taking in,
analyzing, and acting on increasingly broad, deep, and interconnected
types of information from interactions with patients and families. As they
become more sophisticated clinicians, physicians usually progress from
managing information about physical symptoms, to dealing with emotional
affect, to working with the social systems that are involved with patients'
problems.

Medical students, physicians, and other health professionals develop
various degrees of counseling skills based on their interest, training opportunities, and abilities. The learner's interest level influences the amount
of skill acquisition most strongly. The second most influential factor is
the amount and quality of time spent in supervised practice of counseling
skills. The amount of intuitive or learned skill initially shown by a learner
affects the subsequent learning somewhat. Skill level at the beginning of
training predicts the ultimate ability of the practitioner less well, however,
than interest and willingness to work persistently on improving (11).

Systems-oriented counseling assumes that the solution to a problem is
related to the personal interactions around the problem. To facilitate
change, therefore, the physician needs to get a clear picture of the patient's
family system and needs to become involved with the system in a way
that is helpful. The way the patient presents his/her symptoms to the physician, as well as the symptoms themselves, can be used as information
for finding solutions.

Psychosocial as well as physical complaints are key variables. The patient's family members will be called on as assistants to the patient and

the physician in the healing process. Because every problem is perpetuated by an interconnected set of responses by the patient, family, and physician, the problem can potentially be changed by adjusting any of these responses. Using a systemic approach, the physician enters each patient visit expecting to understand the problem in its biopsychosocial context, and feeling confident that a solution will eventually be found. Systemic solutions can range from completely changing some idea, feeling, or behavior to deciding that the current situation with the symptom is the best one for the person and the family right now.

The patient and family will share as much information and will address the problem as fully as is possible for them to do at that point. Some people are able to share and deal with more than others. When using a systemic approach, the clinician takes a neutral, nonblaming stance toward the patient and his/her family. He/she accepts and uses whatever information and way of presenting it that the patient can manage. Unusual ways of presenting problems are viewed as additional information about the patient and the family as they function in the world. The task of the physician is to use all the available information to help the patient and family find a solution to the problem.

Primary care medical practice that includes systems-oriented counseling considers the family during every patient visit. Family members sometimes come into the office to speak for themselves about the problem. For example, an irritated husband may lead off with, "Doc, my wife is acting real odd lately. I want you to find out what's wrong with her." An exasperated wife may introduce her concern with, "He knows he's got to take the medicine to keep his blood pressure down, but I just can't get him to do it like you told him to." Most of the time, however, the clinician will have to probe for the opinions and reactions of other family members.

The systems-oriented individual interview is conducted using skills that help the physician and patient understand each other and form a therapeutic relationship (4,12–14). Combining counseling skills with theories of human functioning in families produces a humanistic complement that can augment the biomedical approach to the practice of medicine.

The clinician conducting a systemic counseling session has four goals:

1. To involve the patient and appropriate family and community members.
2. To explore the problem as fully as possible, given time constraints. Levels to explore for the individual and the family are the biomedical, behavioral, ideational, and emotional.
3. To understand the changes around the problem in each systems level.
4. To design a plan for solving the problem, when appropriate, taking all levels of the system into account.

Achieving and maintaining each goal is necessary to fulfill the next goal. Failure with one goal sabotages success with the others. For example, if the physician does not involve the patient in an acceptable way, he/she will not be able to explore the problem fully because of patient distrust.

As the trust and confidence deepen between physician, patient, and family, open communication allows a freer flow of feelings and information. With more breadth of information about the problem, the changes around the problem can be better understood, and a practical plan for solving the problem can be developed. Skills for achieving each goal of the systemic interview are presented below in an artificially separated manner for purposes of discussion. In actuality each skill is used for multiple purposes throughout the interview.

Skills for Conducting a Systems-oriented Interview

Skills for Goal #1—Involving the Patient

Physicians' verbal and nonverbal responses to patients modify their understanding of the potential for change in the presenting problem. When the physician and patient have good rapport, the potential for healing is greatly enhanced. The opposite is also true, however. If the physician and patient are not responsive to each other, the usefulness of discussion is very limited. When the therapeutic relationship has been compromised, reestablishing rapport takes top priority in subsequent interactions. The skill areas for involving the patient positively are preattending and attending.

Preattending

The most effective preparation for a patient visit enables the clinician to focus completely on the patient and the presenting problem. The ideal environment is safe, private, and comfortable. Pressing physiologic needs (such as going to the bathroom) are met before moving to the next patient. Information from the chart and other sources is best reviewed prior to beginning the visit. Tasks that might interrupt the interview are taken care of, if feasible, and arrangements made to defer them if they cannot be quickly completed. Upon entering the examination room, the physician introduces him/herself to new patients and anyone accompanying them, and asks each person's name if they do not introduce themselves. A non-threatening opening inquiry is, "How did you come to see me today?" With familiar patients the physician may chat briefly about some non-threatening topic before inquiring about the reason for the visit.

Attending

The physician uses verbal and nonverbal openings and responses to join with the patient. Nonverbal means, such as a comfortable degree of eye contact for the patient and a receptive body posture (sitting at the same level as the patient without intervening furniture or fixtures, facing the patient squarely with arms uncrossed, trunk vertical or inclined slightly forward) convey that the physician is listening attentively to the patient with an open mind. During this time, the physician observes the patient's appearance and behavior, making early tentative inferences about energy, tension, mood, and general physical condition. A comment about these observations, e.g., "You look all excited today," is sometimes useful for beginning the interview.

Skills for Goal #2—Exploring the Problem at All Levels

Initiating discussion of the problem

An open question such as "How can I help you today?" invites the patient to focus on his/her concern. This signals the end of the social stage and the beginning of the problem stage of the interview. As the patient begins, the physician encourages a full description of the problem by nonverbal means (nodding) and minimal verbalizations such as "Uh-huh" and "Hmmm." Listening to the patient, the physician maintains a nonjudgmental attitude to understand the problem from the patient's perspective.

Gathering and integrating information

The physician receives and integrates information on three different levels (behavior, emotional, and ideational). To do this, the physician can use declarative or exclamatory responses ("That must have been difficult for you."), as well as questions to facilitate the patient's explanation of the problem.

The clinician uses these statements to feed back the patient's story so that it can be further clarified and expanded. The restatement of the patient's message by the physician allows the patient to understand the physician sees the problem. The feedback statement can include the content of the message, the patient's feelings about the situation, and the meaning of these events to the patient. A useful rule of thumb is for the physician to make at least two statements for each open-ended question asked in the interview.

Open-ended questions are best used early in the visit to avoid premature narrowing of the focus. ("What else is bothering you about this situation?") As the interview proceeds and hypotheses are formed, closed questions become more useful to elicit specific facts and test hypotheses ("I wonder if your headaches have anything to do with the stress of taking care of your elderly mother without any help from your sisters. How much do you think they might be related?").

Avoiding premature closure

Physicians often concentrate on the medical aspects of a problem too early in the interview and steer the patient away from describing what is most important to them. A common predicament for the physician who does this is to complete a biomedical work-up and find him/herself in the uncomfortable position of telling the patient, "I cannot find anything wrong. All the tests are negative." In many cases, the patient's most pressing issue is emotional upset or concern about the meaning of a symptom, whether or not there is a problem that needs biomedical management. ("Does this mean I have cancer? Maybe the doctor just can't find it yet.") If all aspects of the problem are reviewed from the beginning of the physician–patient interaction, a workable solution, including specific rather than vague reassurance, is more likely to be found.

Responding appropriately to feelings and meanings

In responding to feelings and meanings appropriately, the physician listens alertly as the patient tells about his/her concern. The experience of illness is modified as the patient presents it to the clinician. Past experiences with seeking help from physicians or other helpers influence the patient's emotional state, his/her expectations, and his/her behavior in talking to the physician. The physician's responses to the patient's feelings about his/her symptoms and the physician's sharing his/her hypotheses about the problem can help the patient understand the problem in new ways. New understandings suggest possible solutions, as shown in the following example.

PHYSICIAN: When you get the pains in your chest, you feel scared. That keeps you from asking your wife for help because you don't want to upset her.

PATIENT: Hmmm, I think you may be right about that. Maybe she worries more when I don't ask for help than she would if I did ask for help.

The skills for exploring the problem in an individual interview are illustrated in an elaboration of Clinical Example #2. Notice the physician's thinking, listening, and action as she helps the patient tell her story in each step of the interview.

Sue, a 35-year-old single parent, is making her first visit to Dr. W for "a general check-up." The medical intake sheet also states that her two children, Amy, age 10, and Chad, age 7, live with her.

M.D. preattending thinking: This patient has the life stress of being a single parent. She may consider herself finished with the child-bearing years, while she may be starting new primary intimate relationships. This could create a strain between conflicting tasks of the two family life cycle stages.

M.D. preattending behavior: Involve the patient in the interview process by establishing rapport. Social conversation and warm nonverbal contact are called for.

M.D. attending behavior: Dr. W begins the interview by chatting with the patient about the area of the city she lives in, and about her experience of arranging for the appointment. She then prepares to ask the reason for the visit.

M.D. attending thinking: There are already a lot of possibilities, but I will let the patient start in her own way, rather than exploring one of my own early hypotheses.

DR. W: *(M.D. behavior: Open question)* What can I help you with today?

SUE: Well, I haven't had a checkup for three years, and I would like to find out if the pain in my stomach is anything to worry about.

(*M.D. thinking:* Sue may be very worried about the pain.)

DR. W: (*M.D. behavior: Response to feeling*) Tell me more about your concerns.

SUE: Well, I've generally been a healthy person, and I eat well. I get some exercise at the health spa at least twice a week, and I've only been hospitalized twice in my life when my children were born.

(*M.D. thinking:* Sue is telling me she is a responsible, healthy person.)

DR. W: (*M.D. behavior: Response to content*) It sounds like you're taking good care of yourself, and that includes coming in for a checkup.

SUE: Well, I really don't want to end up like my mother when I'm fifty-five, so I thought I'd better come in.

(*M.D. thinking:* Sue is worried about her mother's condition and about herself.)

DR. W: (*M.D. behavior: Minimal verbal facilitation*) Your mother?

SUE: Yes, she just found out that she has breast cancer and is having radiation treatments starting next week. She had a terrible time after the mastectomy, with an infection in the wound, and she got so depressed.

(*M.D. thinking:* This patient's family is stressed by her mother's life-threatening illness and her mother's depressed feelings about the illness.)

DR. W: (*M.D. behavior: Response to feeling*) Sounds like you've been through a lot lately.

SUE: Yes, I guess I have. I hadn't really thought about it. I'm pretty close to my mom, and I hate to see her suffer. I think she's through the tough part now, so I can start thinking about my own life again.

(*M.D. thinking:* The coping strategy in this family is to focus on supporting the person in distress, sometimes at the expense of oneself. Sue is redefining her understanding of the problem as the interview progresses.)

DR. W: (*M.D. behavior: Response to the content and feeling, connecting feelings about mother and patient herself*) You've been so worried about her that you haven't noticed what a strain you've been under.

SUE: Uh-hm. The kids have been a big help to me. They never used to clean up after dinner or do their homework without being told. Now they're doing those things regularly. It seems like they knew that I really needed the help and were able to come through.

(*M.D. thinking:* The children have learned the same coping strategy as mom and grandma.)

DR. W: (*M.D. behavior: Summarize content and feeling, addressing the family as a unit, showing respect and support for the patient*) You're obviously a sensitive family. You noticed your mom's distress over her cancer treatment and felt sad that she was having such a hard time. Your kids seem to have noticed that you needed some extra help and did their best to make life easier for you.

SUE: Yeah, we do stick together. I'm pretty lucky.

(*M.D. thinking:* This coping style has its advantages and disadvantages. Given the circumstances it seems to be fairly functional for this family so far. Although I will continue to watch for detrimental effects of so much focusing on other people's distress, I will support this coping style for now, partly in the interest of establishing rapport.)

DR. W: (*M.D. behavior: Support*) You certainly are.

Interview Monitoring Questions

The physician can monitor his/her thinking during the interview by asking herself several questions periodically. These questions have served the authors well in primary patient care, and family practice residents in training have found them useful. Each highlights an important aspect of the systems-oriented interview.

1. *Managing the interview.* "Am I organizing this interview well?", "Do I know where I want to go next?", "What loose ends need tying down?"

These questions remind the physician to direct the interview appropriately to accomplish its purposes, but not to overcontrol it and omit important patient concerns. In the case example, the physician directed the interview by moving from general open-ended questions to responding to the content, feelings, and meaning of the patient's experience, then to summarizing the "findings." The interview flowed well, with a logical progression toward problem definition and management. At times the physician and patient get "stuck." This can happen when the physician loses his/her neutrality or confidence that he/she and the patient can work together to find solutions to the problem. When this happens, it is useful to take a "time-out" by leaving the room and thinking through the situation or discussing it with a supervisor or colleague.

2. *Focusing on the problem.* "How can I tie this part of the discussion back to the problem?"

The physician connects as much of the elicited information as possible to the problem, keeping in mind that the definition of the problem and the relevance of information changes during the interview. Since information that at first seems tangential sometimes turns out to be critical for understanding the broader aspects of the problem, the clinician temporarily postpones judgment about the pertinence of information. At some point in a narrative that appears to have strayed far afield, the physician redirects the discussion back to problem-related information. If Sue had suddenly begun talking about the weather, for example, the physician could ask, "Is there something about the weather you want me to understand so I can do a better job helping you with your problem?" or she could comment, "I'm having trouble understanding how the weather relates to your problem."

3. *Being confident, expectant, and realistic.* "How likely is it that I can work with this patient to help her solve her problems? How responsible am I feeling to solve her problems myself?"

Ideally the physician conveys confidence that he/she can work with the patient to help solve the patient's problems, while acknowledging that he/she is not responsible for the patient's life course. This balanced stance is difficult for most practitioners, since medical training encourages taking a lot of responsibility for patient's outcomes and provides little training to help patients be more responsible for themselves. The physician's directiveness varies with the aspect of the problem being addressed. Medical recommendations are based heavily on the physician's biomedical training, tempered by his/her understanding of human behavior (for example, prescribing once-a-day medication versus two or three doses a day, to improve informed cooperation with the recommended regimen).

Solutions to patient's life problems are based on particular life situations, and are generated through the doctor–patient relationship. The patient and his/her family are ultimately responsible for using the help from the physician, and the realistic physician expects them to act responsibly. If, in our case example, the physician had tried to take charge of Sue's life inappropriately, she might have given premature advice such as "Sue, just remember you are not your mother. Take your mind off your stomach pain by reading a good book." The physician could have overmedicalized the problem by launching into an elaborate review of systems and a laboratory test work-up. Another inappropriate physician response would have been a misguided intervention like "Sue, I'm going to call your mother and advise her to stop worrying you with her problems."

4. *Being neutral and nonblaming.* "How clearly am I thinking about this patient and the problem?", "How much am I reacting to my own feelings?"

The physician can be more effective when he/she distinguishes his/her own feelings from his/her understanding of an emotionally intense situation for the patient. The physician awareness of his/her own feeling responses to the patient can help in understanding what the patient is experiencing, but unless the physician is careful, he/she can allow his/her feelings about the patient to compromise his/her effectiveness. Discussion groups can help physicians understand their emotional reactions to patients. One such forum is called a Balint group, after the psychiatrist who originated and wrote about them in England (15). Physicians participate in Balint groups in many different countries, and some family practice residency programs conduct them on an ongoing basis (16). Deepening their understanding of their feelings about patients through group discussion often leads physicians to develop more choices for their behavior with patients.

While the physician in our case example imagined herself in Sue's shoes and responded empathetically to her in the interview, she did not let her feelings about her own mother or her own children color her interaction with Sue. The professional stance toward all individuals in the patient's family system is neutral and nonblaming. If the physician began thinking, "I like Sue, but her mother sounds horribly overbearing," she would find it very difficult to avoid taking sides. To minimize this tendency, she could meet with both Sue and her mother to help them work out their differences. Sometimes a second family member will wish to meet with the physician alone for the first encounter to "tell their side" without the other person, who already has a relationship with the doctor, being present. Done judiciously, this may be useful, but if continued it can result in an alternating cycle of "my turn at bat." After one visit alone, both family members can be brought in together and the clear message given that the physician is not going to choose sides.

5. *Understanding the problem as part of the family system.* "Have I explained the family involvement in this problem?"

Physicians can be most effective by using a family-centered approach. If Sue had complained bitterly about another family member, and her physician only explored Sue's feelings about that person, Sue may have returned home saying, "My doctor agrees with me that you are a miserable witch!" If, instead, the physician explored the whole family involvement and then planned to meet with as many family members as possible, she would have had a much better chance to help the family solve the problem.

6. *Intervening with the entire family system.* "How feasible do I think it is for me to work with all members of this family?"

The systems-oriented clinician trusts that everyone in the family will benefit from being involved, at least in the stage when the problem is identified and clarified. The physician in our example kept an open mind about Sue's family, assuming that Sue's mother, ex-husband, and children could all play a role in her symptom. The physician also assumed that she could form a positive alliance with each family member. In cases where the physician feels very negative about one key family member, it is probably best to refer the family for necessary family counseling.

Family Interview Skills

If the problem involves the patient's family, it may not be possible to understand it without seeing and hearing from all members of the family. Skills for exploring the problem in a family interview are discussed below.

Calling a family meeting

In bringing the family together it is important to focus on the problem. People are usually willing to attend a family session if they understand that their point of view will be respected, and that it is needed to help solve the problem. If people think they will be blamed or criticized, they will probably come with great reluctance, if at all. The physician can let family members know that he/she would like to meet with the whole family to get their valuable input to help solve a problem that affects the whole family. Sometimes the patient can bring the family in unassisted. When the patient is unsuccessful or pessimistic about being able to convince the others to come, the physician can obtain permission to phone the family members him/herself and ask them to come.

Exploring the problem in a family meeting

In exploring the problem in a family meeting, the physician reviews the same three levels as in the individual interview—what the family members are thinking, feeling, and doing around the problem. Changes in the family system over the time of the problem are noteworthy, as are disagreements between family members. The physician observes family interactions with respect to the systems characteristics of wholeness, organization, patterning, and evolution. To explore the symptom at the behavioral level, the clinician attempts to define the problem and to track behavioral sequences.

Defining the problem

After the introductory social stage of the family meeting, the physician opens the problem-oriented stage of the interview by asking each member to describe the problem for which the meeting was called, as well as any other problems that they think need to be addressed. Since the goal is to explore and define the problem at the family level, each person is asked to give his/her opinion so that differences in perception are clear from the start. Difficulties in resolving differences can then be identified as part of the problem for the family.

The physician then asks the family to describe a slow-motion picture of the events leading up to the problem, the problem situation itself, and subsequent events since the onset of the problem. Families have difficulty doing this without talking in generalities and giving highly subjective descriptions, as in the following family interview conducted recently by the authors.

The family members are father, mother, 8-year-old daughter (Sheryl), and 8-month-old son (Steven). The interviewers are a family physician (FP) and a family therapist (T).

FP: Can you tell me what you were looking for today?

FATHER: Had no idea.

T: Does anybody have anything they wanted to talk about?

FATHER: I wanted to see if you could improve her health a little. She *(pointing to Mom)* gets nervous—probably from Sheryl—a little bit, and her stomach goes, and she has poor appetite. *(To mother)* What was that in your stomach?

MOTHER: Spasmotic contractions.

FATHER: Yeah, she can't eat regular food.

MOTHER: I get a lot of heartburn and I'm very nauseous.

FATHER: We have steak and she can't eat it. All she has is salad or bread.

T: So you're worried about your wife because she has trouble with her stomach, and it's affected the family to the extent that she has to eat something different than the rest of you?

FATHER: Yeah.

T: How does that affect the meals that you have?

FATHER: Sheryl and I eat like kings. *(Laughter. Everyone looks at Sheryl.)*
T: You get steak and Mom doesn't?
FATHER: I think something can be done about it. She's a healthy girl, still young. *(Gesturing toward Mom)*
T: Have you two talked about this?
FATHER: Yeah, I'm alright if she is.
MOTHER: That's why I've been at the doctor's so much.
T: Were you aware that he was concerned?
MOTHER: He always is.
T: How do you know he's concerned about you?
FATHER: I tell her. *(Laughter)*
T: When do you tell her? *(Silence)*
T: *(to Mom)* Is that what prompted you to come in, in the first place?
MOTHER: I was having terrible pains in my stomach.
FATHER: Yeah, she was even doubled over one time.

The interviewers now know that the mother's symptom prevents her from sharing the same food with Sheryl and father, and that when she complains about the pain, her husband tells her he's concerned and that she should go to the doctor. One hypothesis would be that the mother may not be satisfactorily involved with the father, who has a cross-generational alliance with his daughter. A corollary hypothesis would be that the mother comes to the doctor to get some more caring attention than she gets from her husband.

Another hypothesis would be that the mother and Sheryl are not well connected since the arrival of the new baby 8 months ago, and that there may be subacute hostility in their relationship. The mother might easily remain overinvolved with her infant son in another cross-generational alliance. The problem of Mom's abdominal pain has been redefined during this discussion in terms of family interactions. Among other potentials for adverse outcomes, this situation holds increased risk for incestual interaction between father and daughter, because both of them may feel neglected by mother and could turn to each other to meet their intimacy needs if the dysfunctional alliances persist.

Tracking behavioral sequences

Behavioral sequences are tracked to elucidate the pattern of behavior around the problem that the family is unable to change on their own. This kind of pattern often involves an attempted solution to the original family problem, with the intended solution having now become the problem itself. Changed or changing alliances between family members are often revealed that show how the pattern holds members of the family together. Look for the behavioral sequence in a later segment of the same interview with the family above.

MOTHER: The teacher's on my back. She *(Sheryl)* wasn't in school for a week and the teacher said she's had it with Sheryl. She is distracting everybody.

FP: So the teacher called you?

MOTHER: I had to pick her up because she was staying after school every afternoon. The teacher says she doesn't listen. What can I do?

T: So what did you do?

MOTHER: If she'd just listen, she wouldn't have any problem.

T: So what have you done to remedy the problem?

MOTHER: Well, she hasn't been staying after school anymore, but she is getting bad marks.

FP: So what did you do?

MOTHER: I told her she had to start paying attention, and if she didn't smart up, she'd have to stay back.

FATHER: We took some T.V. away.

T: Did the two of you decide together to take away T.V. privileges?

FATHER: I think in a few years she'll understand that it is bad to stay back.

T: Have you two talked this over?

MOTHER: We've restricted her bicycle.

T: Did you two talk it over?

FATHER: No. She does more of the discipline because I'm not there.

By continuing to ask "what do people do" the physician and therapist found that privileges such as television and bicycle use are restricted by mom and dad. Note that more detailed information is still needed about how this decision is made and carried out to understand the sequence. The parents' answers to questions about whether they talked about the situation strengthens the hypothesis that the parents' communication and negotiation around disciplining Sheryl may be ineffective, keeping Sheryl triangled with her parents.

Examining coalition alignments

The physician explores the emotional aspects of the family system to better understand how emotions are expressed in the family and what functions they serve. The expression of feelings by one individual strongly influences other family members. Like the interrelatedness of other behaviors, expressing one's feelings affects others, and others' behavior affects how one expresses feelings. The patterned system of emotions is key information for the clinician to use in forming hypotheses. One category of questions about the emotional sphere explores coalition alignments and triangles. Such questions include:

- "Who is upset when . . . ?"
- "Who feels more helpless when . . . ?"
- "Who notices first when . . . ?"

Continuing the above case, look for how mother and daughter express their emotions in patterned sequences in the following discussion of Sheryl's school work.

FP: Who gets the most upset about Sheryl?

MOTHER: I think I do.

FP: *(To Sheryl)* So Mom helps you—and what happens?

MOTHER: She just wants me to do the work for her.

SHERYL: I *don't* want her to give me the answers. I just want her to help me, but when she does, she gets too aggravated.

FP: Tell me exactly what happens.

SHERYL: Sometimes I ask her to help and she gets mad and I start to cry. Sometimes I didn't do nothing—like she got mad at me for squeaking the toy, but I wasn't squeaking it, Steven was, but she blames it on me.

FATHER: *(To Mother)* Sheryl really tries to get along with you.

MOTHER: *(To Sheryl)* You don't have to be so sensitive.

Here the mother's pattern appears to be to express her generalized frustration by getting mad at Sheryl, who then cries, which brings the father in to comfort Sheryl. The way feelings are expressed in the family reinforces the cross-generational coalition of father and daughter, and it leaves the mother alone with her frustrations, without a husband ally in the parent generation.

Examining belief systems and explanations

The ideational level is explored by listening for the family's beliefs and for the way the problem is perceived and explained by the family. The clinician needs to know what they think about the cause and cure for the problem, and how they react to each other's beliefs. The words they use to describe the problem often reveal the belief system. For example, in the same case, when discussing discipline:

MOTHER: She listens to her father, not me. I can talk till I'm blue in the face.

FATHER: It's just like when I was in school—a man has more control.

FP: So you, dad, have more control? Does it happen that way when mom tries to discipline when dad's at home?

MOTHER: Oh, yeah, she listens when her father's around. Like in the morning, I say get dressed, get dressed, but then her father speaks up and she gets going.

Here a lack of wholeness is seen in the family's beliefs about discipline. Mother is defined as the primary disciplinarian when father is at work. Yet father is defined, in this traditional family, as having ultimate control in the family. The physician can hypothesize that Sheryl will continue to misbehave with her mother until her parents learn how to work together in disciplining the children. In the following discussion of the mother's abdominal pain, information is obtained about the family's explanations.

FP: How do you folks explain this?

FATHER: She thinks it's nerves.

MOTHER: Yeah, like I told you, Sheryl has trouble in school. Tuesday night I helped her with her homework, and I got so riled up I had pains all night. She brought home a pile of papers with failing grades, and I tried to help her, and she wasn't there, you know?

FATHER: She can't concentrate.

MOTHER: She's very distracted, but yet when he's with her, she can do it at home.

FATHER: I think when she's with someone, she does better. At school there are twenty kids and she gets distracted.

MOTHER: The teacher says she talks too much and is very careless.

FP: So you've got information from the teacher that she has trouble . . . .

Here the abdominal pain symptom is linked strongly with the family's description of the mother's lack of capability with her daughter. One hypothesis about this would be that the mother's powerlessness somehow functions to keep the family together, perhaps because the parents believe that a powerful wife would emasculate her husband.

Family themes can also be revealed by doing and exploring genograms (see Chapter 8 for details). Myths and beliefs over several generations of a family can have pervasive effects on the present situation.

Skills for Goal #3—Understanding Changes Around the Problem

Examining time progression

The patient, the family, and the physician can begin to predict the outcome of tentative plans for the future as they begin to understand changes from the past to the present. Asking the family to classify and compare situations at different times reveals when things were better and worse, and brings out the changes that coincide with the onset of the symptom. In planning for changes in the system, it is useful to use "What if" questions. In this way, the family's fears about change can be discussed and solutions planned to minimize resistance to change.

Personalizing the problem

By this point in the interview, the physician and patient, as well as the family in some cases, have established good rapport and have explored the behavior, feelings, and thinking about the problem. Through discussing interactions around the problem, connections between the symptom and the family system have been revealed. At this point, the clinician summarizes how the patient, the family, and the problem are connected. The strengths and weaknesses of the patient and family for coping with the problem can then be clarified. Thoroughly exploring the symptom and its context provides the basis for the physician and the patient to understand the problem accurately, and sets the stage for initiating an action plan. The skills for planning are described in the next section.

Skills for Goal #4—Taking Action on the Problem

Defining a goal

With information about family resources, the patient and family are asked to define a goal that addresses the problem. The physician gives specific recommendations about the medical treatment of the problem, if needed. For changes in behavior by the patient and the family, it is best for the physician and the family to work together to decide what action they will take. In many cases, the chance to talk over the problem with the physician as an outside facilitator will reveal differences and solutions that the family can address on their own.

Handling disagreement about goals or plans for their implementation

If the family members cannot agree on a goal or on a plan to accomplish the goal, the family probably needs to make a basic change in the way they operate (a second order change). A thorough evaluation of family function would be indicated for such a family. Christie-Seely's adaptation of the McMaster Model of Family Function, called PRACTICE, is a useful tool for this purpose (17,18). A self-report questionnaire, the Family Assessment Device, also could be helpful to the clinician (19).

Intervening to change the family system

Many books detail ways of intervening at different levels of the problems of individuals and families. Because complex systems interventions are beyond the scope of this book, they will not be discussed. Clinicians with more family therapy training than primary care physicians are valuable members of the health care team. They can assist the patient and the family with problems that are beyond the competency, time availability, and interest of most physicians who are not psychiatrists.

Consulting with and referring to family therapists

Unless the physician has advanced psychotherapy training, referring the family that does not respond to straightforward counseling for more intensive and complex therapy is in order. One of the best indicators that the physician needs to refer a family is when the physician feels overwhelmed or persistently confused while seeing the patient or the family. While this may seem obvious, it is nonetheless difficult for many physicians to do something that they think the patient and family will interpret as the physician's rejecting them. If the physician feels defeated and pessimistic when making the referral, the patient and family will sense those feelings and will be unlikely to connect well or at all with the new therapist.

A good referral can be made by saying something like "Well, we've given it a good try, but I think your problem is just too complicated for me to help you with. I know someone who has helped several of my patients with similar problems before. I think he/she may be able to help you with your difficult problem. I'd be glad to arrange an appointment for you, and could go with you for the first visit if you like. How would you like to see him/her?"

Because many patients are more sensitive about psychosocial issues than medical ones, the consultation/referral process for psychotherapy is a bit trickier. The family may or may not be receptive to working on the problem with a family therapist, but if the physician presents the referral in a positive light, the family is more likely to follow through with it. If feasible, the physician may arrange to meet with the family and the new therapist for the first session to facilitate the transition and legitimize the referral in the eyes of the family.

Another factor that complicates the consultation/referral process is the difference in educational background between physicians and family therapists, compared to the more similar training of primary care physicians and other medical specialists. The physician may be uncomfortable sending a patient to someone who works with patients in ways he/she doesn't understand very well. The physician may also have some personal beliefs about psychotherapy that generate ambivalence in his/her referral communications. Counseling, consulting, and referring can all be done most effectively if the physician is aware of some of the hidden aspects of the doctor–patient relationship, which are discussed below.

The Doctor, the Patient, and the Family

Physician–patient relationships are actually multilateral, because both physician and patient live with families, social support groups, and communities. Many pathways of influence and counterinfluence exist in and between these systems. One three-part system is a powerful basic unit in medical care—the *therapeutic triangle*. Most of medical training views the doctor–patient relationship as one-on-one and ignores its social context, producing what has been termed "the illusion of the dyad in medical practice" (10). Most physician interactions with patients involve the patients' family because most patients are so strongly influenced by them.

Just as an individual's life is disrupted by illness, a family's organization is also thrown into disequilibrium. Reorganization can affect family members in positive ways, such as strengthening affectional ties, or in negative ways, such as increasing levels of conflict and precipitating divorce (20, 21). A positive physician–family relationship enables the physician to help the family through the crises of illness. The patient receives optimal treatment when family members can support the program and work through their reactions to the illness.

The therapeutic triangle affects how the physician practices medicine. The patient's family supports or undermines the physician's relationship with the patient. Since medical treatment is usually carried out in the family setting, rather than in the doctor's office, the family can influence the patient's response to treatment in crucial ways. Whether the problem is more medical or more psychosocial, the family plays an important role in the diagnosis, treatment, and resolution of the problem. The physician can often positively affect the family's involvement. If, instead of working solely with a male patient on a weight loss plan, the physician also meets with the patient's wife and engages her in the plan, the patient may have more success with achieving and maintaining weight loss.

The physician–patient relationship can have a strong positive or negative impact on the patient–family relationship. For instance, a female physician related very well with a male patient she saw alone frequently for poorly controlled hypertension. As the patient came to trust the physician, he shared with her information he had never told anyone else—he divulged his problem with alcohol. If the physician continued to meet with him alone to work on the problem, she might weaken the marital relationship, particularly if (as is usually the case) the marriage was already strained. The wife would probably feel hurt and jealous being excluded from such an important facet of her husband's life. Further, she may undermine her husband's efforts to stop drinking unless she is actively included in the treatment efforts. The physician who is aware of the therapeutic triangle will bring the wife into some of the visits.

Physicians who are not careful may wind up undermining rather than strengthening family relationships during stressful periods. If the physician sees someone who has a negative relationship with a significant other person (unresolved conflict), the patient may draw the physician into a supportive alliance with him/her. The physician can derive satisfaction from providing a valued interaction with the patient. If this becomes the patient's major source of positive interaction, however, the physician may feel overburdened with the needs and demands of that patient. Consequently he/she will have less time and energy for the rest of his/her patients, his/her family, and him/herself. If the demands of the physician's patients are not responded to in a realistic way, the clinician may withdraw from his/her own family. The physician who gets in over his/her head with patients moves from the therapeutic triangle to a medical "Bermuda Triangle," where all sorts of strange and unpleasant things happen. The physician who is aware of the therapeutic triangle can maximize the payoff from efforts to benefit patients and their families.

Summary

Primary care physicians work with patients and their families in a privileged relationship, helping them care for illness and maintain health. Skillful interventions using systems-oriented counseling can bring great satisfaction to the physician and considerable advantage to patients. Physicians continue to learn on many levels throughout their careers. This chapter offers some basic knowledge about skills for exploring and working with family systems. These basics can serve as a foundation for more extensive learning about helping families improve their health and functioning.

References

1. Engel GL: The need for a new medical model: A challenge for biomedicine. Science 1977;196:129–136.
2. Crouch MA, McCauley J: Family awareness demonstrated by family practice residents: Physician behavior and patient opinions. J Fam Pract 1985;20:281–284.
3. Crouch MA, McCauley J: Interviewing style and response to family information by family practice residents. Fam Med 1986;18:15–18.
4. Papp P: The Process of Change. New York, Guilford Press, 1983.
5. Carter E, McGoldrick M (eds): The Family Life Cycle: A Framework for Family Therapy. New York, Gardner Press, 1980.
6. Huygen FJA: Family Medicine: The Medical Life of Families. New York, Brunner/Mazel, 1982.
7. Bateson G: Mind and Nature—A Necessary Unity. New York, Bantam Books, 1979.
8. Bateson G: Steps to an Ecology of Mind. New York, Ballantine Books, 1972.
9. Minuchin S: Families and Family Therapy. Cambridge, MA, Harvard University Press, 1974.
10. Doherty W, Baird M: Developmental levels in family-centered medical care. Fam Med 1986; 18:153–156.
11. Gurman AS, Raisen AM: Effective Psychotherapy: A Handbook of Research. New York, Pergamon Press, 1977.
12. Carkhuff RR: The Art of Helping, ed 5. Amherst, MA, Human Resources Development Press, 1984.
13. Haley J: Problem-Solving Therapy. San Francisco, Jossey-Bass, 1976.
14. Minuchin S, Fishman HC: Family Therapy Techniques. Cambridge, MA, Harvard University Press, 1981.
15. Balint M: The Doctor, His Patient, and the Illness, ed 2. New York, Pittman, 1964.
16. Brock CD: Balint group leadership by a family physician in a residency program. Fam Med 1985;17:61–63.
17. Christie-Seely J: Working with the Family in Primary Care: A Systems Approach to Health and Illness. New York, Praeger Publishers, 1984.
18. Miller I, Epstein NB, Bishop DS: The McMaster Family Assessment Device: reliability and validity. J Mar Fam Ther 1985;11:345–356.
19. Epstein NB, Bishop DS: Problem-centered systems therapy of the family, in Gurman AS, Kniskern DP (eds): Handbook of Family Therapy. New York, Brunner/Mazel, 1981, pp 444–482.
20. Bruhn JG: Effects of chronic illness on the family. J Fam Pract 1977;4:1057–1060.
21. Margolin G, Kingsolver K: Disorders of Family relationships, in Blechman, E, Brownell, K (eds): Behavioral Medicine for Women. New York, Pergamon Press, in press.

CHAPTER 8

Using the Genogram (Family Tree) Clinically

Michael A. Crouch and Terry Davis

What Is a Genogram?

The genogram (family tree) is an extraordinarily versatile clinical tool that can help inexperienced clinicians obtain family and social history information from patients more easily. The more experienced the clinician becomes, the more effective and time efficient the genogram is for helping the clinician elicit family information and use it to take good care of patients.

The genogram can be thought of as an X-ray of the family—an "x ray without the roent." It gives the physician and the patient a graphic display of the family, including the family's patterns of illness and psychosocial problems. When patients see the constellations of family disease and problems highlighted on the family tree, they appear to take them more seriously, as if realizing their implications for the first time. The sedentary, overweight, hypertensive, diabetic, cigarette-smoking man whose genogram is shown in Figure 8.1 began to acknowledge the likely consequences of his life-style and poor compliance with his medical regimen after seeing his genogram drawn out. The dramatic pattern of early coronary heart disease is more vivid in graphic form.

The genogram often reveals family skeletons (e.g., an illegitimate child), dislocated families (e.g., with a disowned or runaway child), osteoporotic families vulnerable to stress fracture (e.g., a distant marital relationship nearing the empty nest phase of the life cycle), and families with compound fractures (multiple divorces and remarriages). The physician does not have to *do* anything with this information except record it and keep it in mind when he/she sees family members in the future. It may or may not ever be directly relevant to patient care, but if it is not known, its relevance cannot be judged. Depending on the patient, the physician, and the circumstances of the visit (including how busy the physician is), some family information will suggest preventive or therapeutic intervention by the physician and/or referral to other community resources. For example, eliciting a family history of spouse abuse may open the door for a female

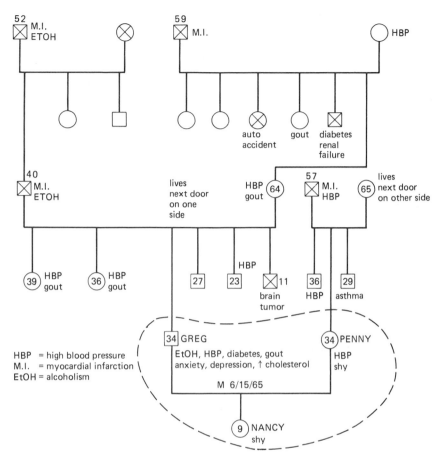

FIGURE 8.1.   Family illness patterns as revealed in a genogram.

patient to tell the physician that her husband has been beating her for
several months. The physician can then do brief supportive counseling
and put the woman in touch with the nearest shelter for battered women.

The process of the physician and the patient drawing the family tree
together facilitates the doctor–patient–family relationship in several ways.
Asking about family information in a structured, matter-of-fact way helps
the interviewer remain objective and reduces physician discomfort when
inquiring about sensitive issues like divorce. When the physician is comfortable with his/her questioning, the genogram seems to foster honesty
by lowering the patient's resistance to talking about embarassing or painful
matters, such as alcoholism and sexual abuse. Sharing family information
with the physician often builds rapport and trust more quickly than usual.

For anxious patients who come in to the doctor in some degree of crisis,
doing a genogram has a nonspecific calming effect. Asking patients factual

questions about their families invites them to move into a rational thinking mode, and encourages them to be less governed by the intense feelings that are dominating their lives at that point. When patients' thoughts and communications are scattered and irrational, focusing on the facts of their families usually helps them concentrate on reality better, allowing them to begin to deal with their problems in a constructive way.

Historical Perspective

The genogram is a modification of the genealogical family tree and the genetic pedigree. The abbreviated version, the "skeletal" genogram, was first described in 1975 (1). Since then several variations in the basic technique have been proposed for doing genograms and using them in patient care (2–9). The first author began doing genograms early in his family

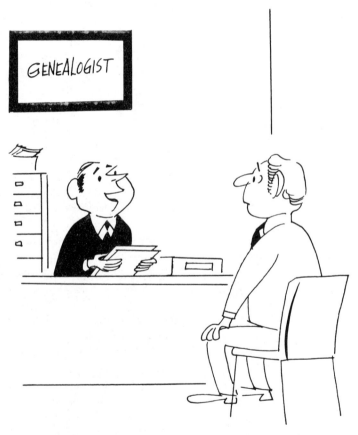

"Shall I continue searching your family tree? I just found one of your relatives hanging from one."

practice residency. He found them to be helpful so often that he almost always gets a genogram as part of his initial evaluation of a new patient. The second author, an experienced psychotherapist, began doing genograms relatively recently. She has been particularly impressed with how much family information can be gotten in a very short time with the genogram, and how quickly she was able to incorporate the genogram into her assessment routine.

This chapter will introduce the genogram technique and discuss how it can be used. Major emphasis will be placed on using the genogram routinely with new patients, and on using it to evaluate and manage puzzling, complicated, or difficult patients. After reading this chapter and doing the learning exercises, you should be able to:

1. Conduct a brief genogram interview, eliciting and recording on a skeletal genogram the basic information about important events and serious illnesses in three generations of a patient's family.
2. Discuss associated patterns of emotional intensity and illness seen in genograms of patient families.

Why Not Do Genograms?

Despite being promoted for the past 5 years, the genogram is not yet widely used in medical settings. Doing a "skeletal" genogram takes 5 to 20 minutes (4,5), time that the busy and stressed clinician may be reluctant to commit to an unfamiliar approach for getting and storing clinical information. A sense of time urgency pushes the clinician to take care of business in a straightforward, no-frills manner much of the time. The authors believe that doing genograms, while taking a little more time in the short run, will actually save time in the long run.

Reviewing the information on the family tree can obviate the need to repeatedly inquire about family history that is forgotten after each visit unless it is recorded somewhere in the chart in retrievable form (10). Often the genogram yields important clues that allow the physician to hone right in on the problem, rather than spending a lot of time going through laundry lists of symptoms. This is particularly true for familial problems that often present in vague ways, such as depression and anxiety disorders (11,12). Anytime the patient is admitted to the hospital, the family history can be extracted easily from the genogram, and kept in mind during diagnostic work-ups and illness management.

For the physician in training, learning to do genograms requires more knowledge and skills to be mastered, on top of the overwhelming amount already expected of the competent physician. Unless the physician trainee decides that the payoff may be worth the effort, dealing with family history and other family matters tends to get squashed under the weight of other higher priorities. More important than saving time, doing a genogram can improve the quality of care given to the patient.

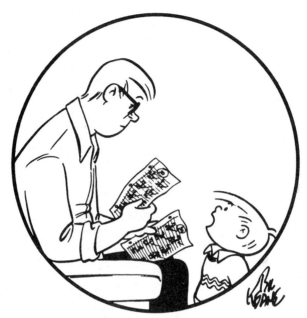

"Miss Johnson thinks she knows my trouble.
What does 'hereditary' mean?"

Many physicians question how appropriate it is for them to venture into the family area, invited or not. Family physicians especially risk biting off more than they can chew and digest. Psychosocial areas seem to be easier for many physicians to resist tackling, perhaps because they are seen as somehow being outside the legitimate purvey of the physician, even if they do strongly affect health and illness (13).

Another reason genograms are avoided is that it is sometimes difficult to decide how to use family tree information to help patients and their families. It is easy to feel overwhelmed by the volume and nature of the data and confused about what to do with it, especially when seeing families like the one in Figure 8.1 with tangled patterns of, for example, heart disease, cancer, alcoholism, diabetes, and depression. When a family is this complicated, the patient is usually confused about his/her problems also. Getting the facts of the family can help the patient and physician pick a place to start to work on a manageable part of a complicated situation.

How to Do a Skeletal Genogram

When a physician sees a new patient, the chief complaint, history of present illness, past medical history, and review of systems take precedence in the interview. After that information is obtained, the clinician traditionally elicits family history and social history and records the information

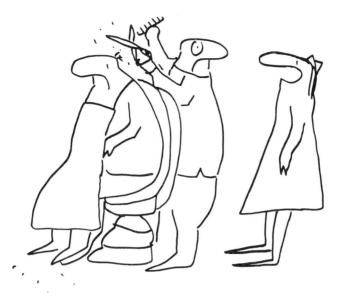

"It may not be my place to say this, Dr. Winkle, but I feel
a general practitioner should establish where his boundaries
are."

in prose form. The genogram is a useful tool for eliciting family and social
history and recording it in a alternative graphic format that highlights patterns of illness and dysfunction in families.

The symbols shown in Figure 8.2 are the ones the authors use for the
genogram. Others use somewhat different notations. Most of these symbols
agree with McGoldrick and Gerson's recently proposed standard set of
genogram symbols (9). For the skeletal genogram, the basic information
includes:

- The sex and approximate age of each family member. For an adult
  patient, this information is obtained for current and past marital partners, children, parents, and grandparents. Information about deceased
  members is often especially useful (e.g., age at death and cause of
  death).
- Serious physical and mental health problems for each family member.
  Specific inquiry is desirable for heart disease, high blood pressure, diabetes, stroke, cancer, nerve problems, depression, alcoholism, and
  suicide.

When doing a genogram, the information is easy to decipher later if
you:

- Indicate the identified patient with a doubly outlined circle or square.
- Place the "clinical nuclear family" roughly in the middle of the diagram,
  with previous marriages off to the right and left.

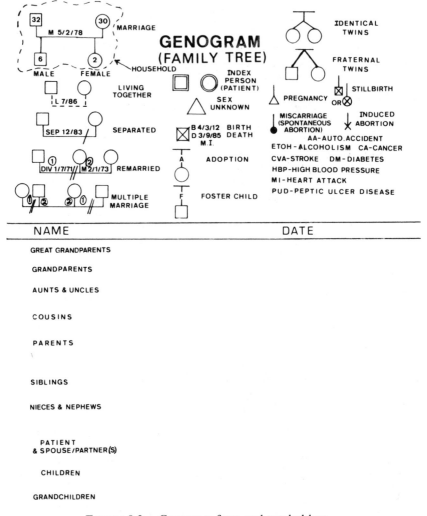

FIGURE 8.2.   Genogram form and symbol key.

- Place siblings in chronological order, unless they are from multiple marriages.
- Offset index patient, spouse(s), and ancestors a little below their siblings.
- Indicate exact age (if known) inside the person's symbol, with date of birth alongside, or indicate approximate ages relative to the patient as $+4$, -3, etc. inside or alongside the circle or square that symbolizes the person.
- Indicate death by crossing through the person's symbol; add date died beside, and age at death inside or alongside the person's symbol.

- Indicate separation with single slash, divorce with two slashes across marriage line.
- Number marriages for spouses, with dates of marriage, separation, and divorce.
- Indicate remarriage to same person with multiple marriage lines.
- Enclose current household members with an interrupted line (dashes).
- Try to keep members of the same generation on the same horizontal level for each branch of the family.

How to Use Genograms in Routine Patient Care

One way to use the genogram is to routinely fill one out on most new patients. A "bare bones" genogram for a family with few members can be drawn in less than 5 minutes on a sheet of paper, or a special form such as the one in Figure 8.2. To fit a genogram on a page this size, make each person's circle or square about 6 to 8 millimeters in diameter and print small. The genogram can be conveniently used if placed at or near the front of the chart—opposite or just under the problem list, for example. One genogram can be done for the first member of each family to be seen, and copies made for the chart of each other family member receiving care in that setting.

Learning Exercise #1: Pregnant and Anxious

The genogram in Figure 8.3 is that of a young woman the first author saw initially for pregnancy care. Before reading the following section, take a minute or two to scan the genogram. Ask yourself, How could the information on this genogram help the physician take good care of the patient?

Jane's only biologic sibling died soon after birth from a neural tube defect 2 years before Jane was born. This raises two important considerations for her care. First, she will probably be much more anxious than the average first-time mother about the normalcy of her baby, and may need more reassurance than usual on this point. Second, because her baby is at increased risk for having a neural tube defect, a screening amniocentesis is indicated.

Social support is another area for concern with this patient. She is now pregnant by either her ex-husband, whom she had been dating until right around the probable time of conception, or by her boyfriend, whom she began seeing around that time also. She was raised by her strict Baptist grandparents. Her grandmother has fortunately been supportive despite the awkward circumstances. Without a resident father figure, parenting will be more stressful for Jane, particularly when stress increases (e.g., when the baby gets sick).

Learning Exercise #2: An Intense Family Practice Resident

A family practice resident's genogram is shown in Figure 8.4. Before reading the material below, scan the genogram briefly. What health prob-

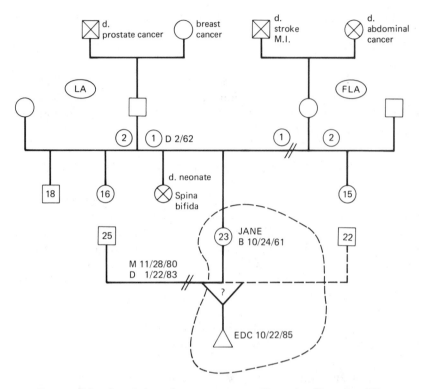

FIGURE 8.3.   Jane's bare bones genogram (Learning Exercise #1).

lems would this physician be vulnerable to under conditions of increased stress?

The most striking patterns in Dr. X's family are those of heart disease, peptic ulcer disease, and alcoholism. While he was chief resident during the third year of his residency, Dr. X experienced multiple episodes of gastric distress, relieved by antacids. He exhibits many of the features of coronary-prone (Type A) behavior. Through family-oriented counseling he realized that, despite sound dietary and exercise habits, he would probably be at increased risk for coronary heart disease in his middle-age years, unless he modified how he handled stress (14). He also identified strong family emotional patterns that appeared to be connected to the illness patterns, and he made substantial progress with changing how he responded to stressful situations. His gastrointestinal symptoms ceased, and his general functioning improved markedly, both personally and professionally.

Learning Exercise #3: Somatization and Loss

The genogram in Figure 8.5 is that of a 7-year-old girl who was referred by a family practice resident to the second author for help with persistent

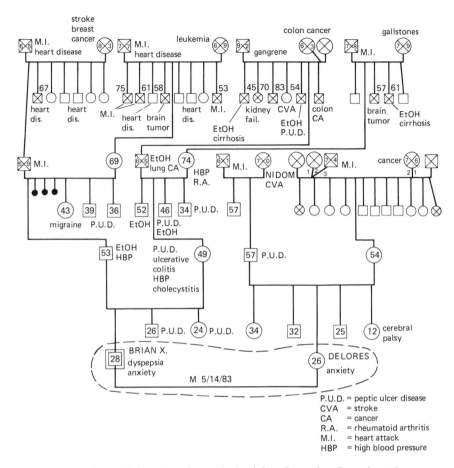

FIGURE 8.4.   Brian X, an intense physician (Learning Exercise #2).

constipation. Before reading the following section, scan the genogram, asking yourself how it could be useful to you as the physician. Then look at it again and think about how it could be useful to a behavioral consultant.

Anna was born with a congenital heart problem (atrial septal defect), which concerned her parents and physicians greatly. She was referred to the behavioral scientist because she was having frequent abdominal pain and had not had an unassisted bowel movement in 6 weeks. She had missed a lot of school. The parents and physicians had tried everything they could think of short of hospitalization. The focus had been mostly on her gastrointestinal system, and some residents were suggesting that she undergo an extensive diagnostic work-up.

   The consultant's objective in doing Anna's genogram was to understand Anna and her symptoms better by seeing what had been happening in the family. She interviewed Anna first, then talked with her mother with Anna in the room to fill in dates and other details. The genogram helped her get important details quickly

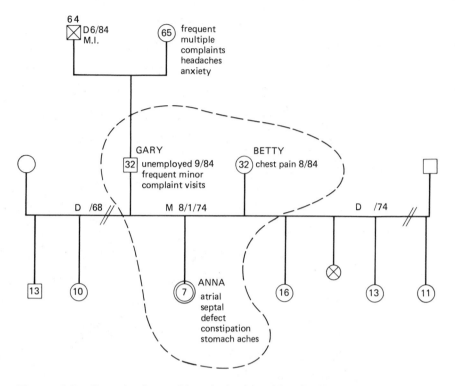

FIGURE 8.5. Somatization and loss in Anna and her family (Learning Exercise #3).

and organize them in a useful manner. The broad questions to be investigated were:

- What's going on with Anna and with her family?
- What bigger picture do her symptoms fit into?

The resident had gotten little family history, and the information he had elicited had not been organized so that it helped him understand the situation.

Anna's stomach aches began in August around the time school started. The genogram shows that Anna's paternal grandfather died of a heart attack 2 months earlier, in June. Anna and her mother had found him dead in the bathroom. Anna was very attached to her grandfather and felt great sadness after his death. Betty, Anna's mother, began having chest pain in August and was taken to the hospital, afraid she was having a heart attack too. The genogram indicates that somatization is a family pattern of responding to stress, with Anna's father, mother, and paternal grandmother all visiting physicians frequently with vague somatic complaints in times of stress. In the interview, the mother stated that Anna was a very special child, the only child of the second marriage for her middle-age parents.

The consultant talked to Anna about her feelings of sadness and anger, and she told Anna that her stomach was pretty smart, that it was saying "I feel something unpleasant. A lot has been going on here." The genogram helped the consultant see the dynamics behind the school avoidance in this child whose medical problems amplified everyone's anxiety. Upon questioning Betty reported that Anna had not been going to school much of the time, and that she got called to pick Anna up on the days she did go. The school, as well as the parents, overresponded to Anna's symptoms. By talking and playing with Anna, the consultant discovered that she was afraid of her mother's potential for having a heart attack, and was scared about her own heart condition.

Treatment focused on dealing with Anna's fear directly instead of her stomach. Together with the resident, Anna's heart condition and Betty's health were discussed with Anna and Betty in great detail. The resident drew Anna's heart and explained the problem she had and answered all her questions. He explained her mother's high blood pressure and stress briefly in age-appropriate terms. Betty was prompted to tell Anna how she was taking better care of her health. In a private session with Anna, the consultant told her that she thought Anna's stomach aches were her sign of distress and fear, and that it might be easier on her stomach if she expressed her feelings more openly. Because she liked to draw, she was encouraged to draw when she felt bad, and to tell her mother about her scary feelings. In a joint session with Anna and her mother, a plan was formulated for leaving her at school unless she was clearly ill in a different way than before. Strategies were developed for Anna's dealing with her fear at school (get a hug from a teacher, for example). The mother was also encouraged to listen to Anna's scary feelings.

Clinicians are aided by the specific details and by the big picture of the family and social situation that the genogram portrays graphically. In this case the genogram helped the behavioral scientist, the resident physician, Anna, and her mother to arrive at a shared understanding of the problem and to solve Anna's problem with constipation and stomach aches. She has done well for over a year since her last session with the behavioral scientist.

Uses of the Genogram

If the clinician scans the genogram for 30 seconds before seeing the patient/client, the information on it can be used to:

- Allow the regular care provider to quickly review the family situation (e.g., second marriage, two of three children born into previous marriages).
- Allow a nonregular care provider to quickly get a sense of the family, improving continuity and comprehensiveness of care (e.g., strong history of anxiety disorders and somatization).
- Build rapport by using the family members' first names.
- Identify significant illness risk factors (e.g., family history of diabetes in an overweight patient).
- Raise the diagnostic index of suspicion. May indicate screening for an individual at high risk (e.g., mammogram with family history of breast cancer).

- Pave the way for sustained patient education about life-style, motivating the patient to make changes (e.g., encouraging smoking cessation with family history of emphysema or lung cancer).
- Demonstrate the clinician's belief that family matters are an important part of an individual's overall health picture (e.g., marital satisfaction).
- Legitimize future discussion of family matters (e.g., problem with a child).
- Allow the patient's family concerns to emerge more quickly than they would otherwise tend to (e.g., erectile dysfunction, soon after it first occurs, rather than after it becomes more resistant to treatment).
- Locate the family in the life cycle, and highlight critical events (15).
- Normalize anxiety related to difficult stages and transitions of the life cycle so that the patient understands his/her distress to be a normal response to a universal stressor (e.g., middle-age adults considering putting their elderly mother in a nursing home).
- Anticipate trouble with future life cycle transitions (e.g., discuss adolescent sexuality and contraception with preadolescents in a family with a tradition of teenage pregnancy).

Learning Exercise #4: Pregnant and Seropositive for Syphilis

The only way to learn whether the genogram could be useful to you as a clinician is to do them with a number of patients and see what you think. To get you started, here is a written summary of the facts about the family of an actual patient the first author saw recently (names changed for anonymity).

Dawn R, an 18-year-old white female, pregnant for the first time, came to the Family Practice Center for prenatal care in December 1985, at about 10 weeks gestation. She was asymptomatic. (Her past medical history will be discussed later.) Her physical examination revealed a uterine size compatible with her menstrual dates, and was otherwise unremarkable.

On a sheet of typing or notebook paper *draw the patient's skeletal genogram,* using the following information and the symbol key in Figure 8.2.

Dawn was born February 28, 1967, the second of four children. She married her husband John in August, 1985. It was the first marriage for Dawn and the second marriage for John, who is 23 years old. John was previously married to Brenda S, from whom he separated on January 8, 1983, and divorced in January, 1984, because of her infidelity. He and Brenda had a son, Randall, born August 2, 1983 (after they had separated), who has been healthy. Brenda has since remarried and has no contact with John.

Dawn has brothers ages 20 (Billy) and 14 (Danny), and a 13-year-old sister (Crystal), all without any serious health problems. Her mother, Mary, age 38, had a duodenal ulcer at age 17; she has high blood pressure, as do two maternal uncles, ages 35 and 30, and the 60-year-old maternal grandmother, Pearl. Dawn's maternal grandfather, Robert, died in 1966 from an oil field injury. Her 43-year-old father,

Dean, spent about 6 months in a hospital with a nervous breakdown, beginning immediately after Dawn's birth. Dean's parents were divorced when he was 2 years old, and he was raised by his maternal grandmother from that point on. Dean has one older brother, age 48, and a half brother age 27 and a half sister age 24, by his mother's second marriage. Dawn's paternal grandfather, Jim, died in 1975 of unknown cause, when Dawn was 8 years old. Her paternal grandmother, Ruth, had a heart attack in 1981.

Look over the genogram you have drawn, and answer these questions:

- What susceptibilities to illness does Dawn's genogram show?
- What psychosocial or emotional patterns are red flags signaling potential problems for Dawn in the future?

The author drew Dawn's genogram as it is shown in Figure 8.6. It isn't important that your drawing be exactly the same, but that it legibly portray

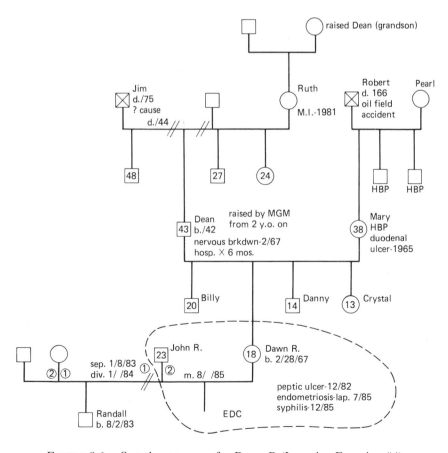

FIGURE 8.6. Sample genogram for Dawn R (Learning Exercise #4).

the people, relationships, and other information accurately. Based on known familial illness patterns and Dawn's family history, she is at increased risk for high blood pressure, peptic ulcer disease, and mental illness (11,12,16,17). She and her family members would be expected to be relatively vulnerable to dysfunction under increased stress.

Dawn's medical history was noteworthy for peptic ulcer disease diagnosed in December, 1982, and endometriosis diagnosed by laparoscopy in July, 1985. She denied any history of veneral disease. She related to the physician comfortably, with good eye contact, and responded articulately to questions. She wore very heavy facial makeup, which often indicates marginal emotional stability.

When her prenatal lab work returned, the serum test for syphilis (RPR) and a confirmatory fluorescent treponemal antibody absorption test (FTA-ABS) were both positive, but a third test, the microhemagglutinin antibody to *Treponema pallidum* (MHATP), was negative. Dawn and John both continued to deny any sexual contact with anyone else, except for John's remote contact with his ex-wife almost 3 years previously. Each of two injections of benzathine penicillin 2 weeks apart was followed by a high fever (Jarisch-Herxheimer reaction versus drug reaction). When John's syphilis serology came back negative, and Dawn continued to steadfastly deny any extramarital intercourse, the diagnostic assessment remained muddled. While the initial test results may have been invalid, a repeat RPR was positive to eight dilutions, indicating a high likelihood of syphilis.

The author will follow Dawn more closely than usual during and after her pregnancy to monitor her emotional coping and watch for other problems. She may be particularly vulnerable to preeclampsia and postpartum depression. Her weight gain so far has been suboptimal despite reported adequate food intake. The confusing syphilis situation continues to stir up anxiety in the couple and the extended families.

Elaborating the Skeletal Genogram

The genogram technique is paradoxical, in that it is both highly structured and very flexible. Since the genogram is not based on any particular theory or approach, it may be used by care providers with various theoretical and clinical approaches. In terms of the personality dimensions characterized by Meyers (18), the genogram can be used comfortably by either the person who gathers and processes data intuitively, or the person who has a more concrete "sensing" approach to data gathering. Both factual cognitive data and subjective emotional information can be easily obtained by probing in areas relevant to the patient's problems. Information from the family tree can be expanded and clues followed up on with straightforward interviewing, or by using supplementary techniques such as the Family Circle (19).

One theoretical-clinical "school" uses the genogram as the main way of gathering information and subsequently working with individuals and families. Multigenerational (Bowen) family systems theory asserts that present patterns of illness and coping with illness stem from patterns in the past (3). Specifically, genetic predispositions interact with life experiences to produce illness in individuals and emotional patterns in families. Illness experiences influence, and are influenced by, the emotional patterns in families.

Family members cope with illness in ways related to how previous generations adapted to members' being ill. Ways of coping with illness include denying its seriousness or existence, being strong, avoiding the ill person, becoming physically ill, and turning to religion or other support systems. Family roles that may shift in response to illness include functional ones such as breadwinner, head of household, and caretaker, as well as less functional ones like family scapegoat and the sick role. Changes in roles following serious illness (e.g., a heart attack) are accompanied by intense feelings of frustration, resentment, and fear of death and dying. As with other emotional patterns, there is a strong tendency for past patterns of coping with illness to recur in succeeding generations. The genogram is well-suited for detecting and clarifying such patterns.

In trying to make sense out of chaotic information the genogram can be used to focus sharply on certain patterns for particular purposes. Chronic illness can be managed better, for example, by getting additional family information to flesh out the skeletal genogram. Elaboration of the skeletal genogram is useful with puzzling, complicated, or difficult patients when:

- Management of a disease or illness is unsatisfactory, and where the reasons are poorly understood or suspected to be related to family matters.
- The patient is disabled or dysfunctional out of proportion to the apparent severity of the disease.
- Serious emotional, behavioral, or physical problems begin or worsen in any family member. The family may present in crisis with such problems.

Gathering expanded genogram information can:

- Give a broader picture of the patient's problems (e.g., daily use of marijuana in a young married woman whose father was alcoholic).
- Estimate a patient's prognosis (e.g., somatization and depression in a 42-year-old woman, two of whose siblings committed suicide).
- Allow a more realistic appraisal of physician and patient goals (establishing a realistic therapeutic plan with the patient in Learning Exercise #4). Decreases doctor and patient frustration by establishing clear boundaries, realistic expectations, and a verbal or written contract spelling out therapeutic goals and responsibilities of the patient and physician.

- Suggest alternate management strategies (e.g., referral to Alcoholics Anonymous, Al-Anon, Al-a-Teen, or Adult Children of Alcoholics).
- Lessen the patients' anxiety by getting them to think about the facts of their families, and by encouraging patients to shift somewhat away from being preoccupied with negative feelings.

To expand the skeletal genogram with chronic illness or disability in mind, some important details to pursue are:

- The dates of onset and diagnosis of serious chronic illnesses.
- The overall course of the illnesses and timing of exacerbations.
- The personal relationships and overall life course of the ill person.
- Who did most of the caretaking for the ill member, for how long, how well, with what attitude about it, with what degree of personal sacrifice, and with what effects on his/her other personal relationships and general functioning.

When more detailed genogram information is being recorded, a larger size paper is needed. A pad of blank paper about 24 by 36 inches works very well for drawing the genograms of occasional families with whom the clinician decides to work more intensively to try to get better results. If the family is seen more than once or twice, the first draft usually becomes very messy, with multiple changes and additions as the family finds out more about its distant members. A redraft that clearly presents the updated facts is easier to work with if the clinician plans to continue seeing the family.

The facts about chronic illness or disability in the family may be used to better understand how the family is handling the situation now, and how it will probably cope in the future, unless something changes. An example of a difficult long-term situation is the "keeper syndrome" (20). As parents age or get sick, someone is elected to the caretaker role. Caretakers usually adopt the role with mixed feelings, which generate conflict (open or submerged) that contributes to health problems, such as headache and depression. The clinician who is aware of the high risk nature of this role can sometimes prevent some of its negative effects by exploring the caretaker's thoughts and feelings and helping him/her negotiate an equitable cooperative arrangement with other relatives.

Often a family that is having difficulty adjusting to chronic illness is repeating a maladaptive pattern from previous generations. If this can be discovered, and clarified with the family, they may then choose between continuing this pattern and pursuing alternatives that promote outcomes that the family prefers. When illness is life-threatening, maladaptive patterns are more rigid and difficult to change. Family members who are acting based on survival urges can seldom calmly analyze and modify their actions without help from a more objective outside party. If the physician is prepared and willing to do so, he/she can help people change maladaptive patterns, like a coach helps athletes get rid of habits that impair performance.

Learning Exercise #5: Your Own Family

The family that you know the most about is your own. The value of using the genogram to learn about families is probably best appreciated by doing your own genogram. If you have not already done so, draw your genogram before reading the next chapter, using the key in Figure 8.2 as necessary. After you have finished it, examine it with these questions in mind:

- What patterns of "physical" illness and disease appear in the various branches of my family?
- What emotional patterns and "mental" illnesses appear?
- Where do I fit into the family patterns in the past? Now? In the future?
- What family patterns am I involved in that have negative implications for my long-term health and functioning and for my family?

Save your genogram and reexamine it after reading the following chapter, in which the first author presents his own family and discusses the benefits to be gained by working on one's own family issues.

Summary

In this chapter, the authors presented the genogram (family tree) as a practical technique for promoting family-oriented care in both training and community practice settings. It can help the clinician take good care of people by:

- Integrating data on the physical and mental aspects of health and illness. (This information is dichotomized in written histories and notes.)
- Graphically displaying multigenerational patterns of illness and dysfunction, for the clinician to use as time, interest, and skills permit.

References

1. Cormack JJ: Family portraits—a method of recording family history. J Roy Coll Gen Pract 1975;25:520.
2. Guerin PJ, Pendagast EG: Evaluation of family system and genogram, in Guerin PJ (ed): Family Therapy: Theory and Practice. New York, Gardner Press, 1976, pp 450–464.
3. Bowen M: Family Therapy in Clinical Practice. New York, Jason Aronson, 1982.
4. Jolly W, Froom J, Rosen MG: The genogram. J Fam Pract 1980;10:251.
5. Rogers J, Durkin M: The semi-structured genogram interview: I. Protocol. II. Evaluation. Fam Syst Med 1984;2(2):176–187.

6. Mullins HC: Collecting and recording family data: The genogram, in Christie-Seely J (ed): Working with Families in Primary Care. New York, Praeger, 1984, pp 179–191.
7. Kramer JR: Family Interfaces: Transgenerational Patterns. New York, Brunner/Mazel, 1985.
8. Sawa R: Family Dynamics for Physicians: A Guide to Assessment and Treatment. Lewiston, NY, Edward Mellen, 1985.
9. McGoldrick M, Gerson R: Genograms in Family Assessment. New York, Norton, 1985.
10. Crouch MA, Thiedke C: Documentation of family health history in the outpatient medical record. J Fam Pract 1986;22:169–174.
11. Crowe RR, Pauls DL, Slymen DJ, Noyes R: A family study of anxiety neurosis. Arch Gen Psychiatry 1980;37:77–79.
12. Jakimow-Venulet B: Hereditary factors in the pathogenesis of affective illness. Br J Psychiatry 1981;138:450.
13. McDaniel SH, Amos S: The risk of change: Teaching the family as the unit of care. Fam Syst Med 1983;1(2);17.
14. Ottman R, Gabrielli C, et al: Family history as an independent risk factor for coronary heart disease. J Am Coll Cardiol 1984;4:793–801.
15. Medalie JH: The family life cycle and its implications for family practice. J Fam Pract 1979;9:47.
16. Zinner SH, Levy PS, Kass EH: Familial aggregation of blood pressure in childhood. N Engl J Med 1971;284:401.
17. Evans DAP: Genetic factors in the etiology of peptic ulcer. Gastroenterology 1961;40:371.
18. Meyers IB: Introduction to Type. Gainesville, FL, Center for Applications of Psychological Type, 1976.
19. Thrower SM, Bruce WE, Walton RF: The family circle method: Integrating family systems concepts in family medicine. J Fam Pract 1982;15:451–457.
20. Banahan BF: The keeper syndrome. Paper presented at the 15th Annual Spring Conference of the Society of Teachers of Family Medicine, Boston, May 3, 1982.

CHAPTER 9

Working with One's Own Family Issues: A Path for Professional Development

Michael A. Crouch

The complex interactions in patients' family systems, and in the therapeutic system that includes the family and the clinician, have been extensively described and analyzed in the literature (1–9). Less attention has been devoted to how issues related to the clinician's nuclear family (10,11) and family of origin (12–14) influence health care and medical education. As the sketch on page 194 shows, every clinical interaction involves the family backgrounds of the clinician and the patient, even though both parties are seldom aware of these dynamics.

Shortly after becoming a faculty member in a family practice residency program, I began a part-time 2-year training program in family therapy, hoping to learn approaches and techniques that could be adapted for use by a busy family physician. The conceptual framework taught in the program was Bowen Family Systems Theory, and I quickly discovered this meant that the training would compel me to examine my relationship with my family to a greater extent than I ever had before.

Learning about myself and my family in this way has been the most valuable educational experience of my life. In this chapter I will discuss the family systems theory that I have found to be most applicable for me as a physician. I will also discuss some of the work I have done on my own family issues, and explain how I have benefited from understanding my family better.

After examining your own genogram (see Learning Exercise #5 in Chapter 8) and reading this chapter, you should be able to:

1. Identify any patterns of illness in your family. What are the implications of these patterns for your health, your health habits, and your life-style?
2. Describe the major emotional patterns, the general level of differentiation, and the level of chronic anxiety in your family.
3. Describe how your family patterns could affect your effectiveness as a physician. What kinds of patients would you be most likely to have difficulty with?

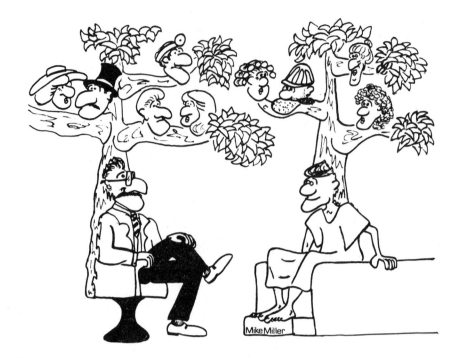

Bowen Family Systems Theory

Bowen Family Systems Theory, developed by psychiatrist Murray Bowen, considers human behavior from a broad multigenerational perspective, focusing on patterns of emotional process over several generations of a given family (15,16). Bowen Theory holds that most serious human problems stem from difficulty coordinating higher functions of the cerebral cortex (rational intellect) with the workings of the evolutionarily older areas of the brain (especially emotions) (17,18). Under stress, the older areas, which have stimulated the reproduction and sustained the survival of the human species, tend to influence behavior more strongly than the higher areas. High stress emotions include anger and fear. A person who acts congruently with these emotions, without overriding dysfunctional behavioral urges with rational thoughts, tends to avoid or attack the stressful situation (the basic biologic "flight or fight" response).

The key concept of Bowen Theory is emotional-intellectual maturity, also termed definition of self, or differentiation. The well-differentiated individual is able to:

1. Think for him/herself.
2. Hold values and goals consistent with self-fulfillment and health.
3. Act responsibly in accordance with values and goals.
4. Relate to others with an appropriate amount of emotional closeness.

5. Distinguish rational considerations from emotional closeness.
6. Base important decisions on mainly rational grounds, in the face of conflicting emotional urges that have counterproductive implications.

Persons with a low level of self-definition are not very autonomous. Their values and goals have been mostly absorbed uncritically from influential others (parents, friends, spouse, church), and some of the values and goals may be mutually incompatible. Some thoughts and feelings blur together almost indistinguishably. Other thoughts and feelings are rigidly compartmentalized, separated so much that they cannot be compared and integrated reasonably. Decision making is dominated by intense feelings and/or sterile rationalization.

Poorly differentiated individuals tend strongly toward excessive or inappropriate emotional involvement (fusion) with others. Emotional fusion can be expressed as mutual dependency, conflict, distance, and illness symptoms. Distance, geographic or psychological, does not resolve emotional fusion. The intensity between parents and their children may appear to abate as the children become adults, but fusion reemerges in the young adults' relationships with their spouses and children. Great distance between generations (emotional cutoff) may produce as much chronic anxiety as conflict does. Chronic anxiety appears to play an important role in the development and course of many illnesses by impairing the immune and other physiologic systems (19,20).

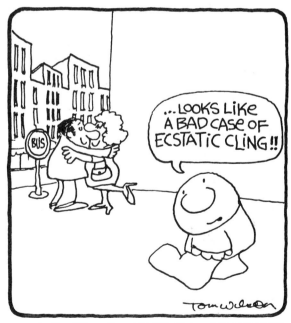

ZIGGY, by Tom Wilson. Copyright 1984, Universal Press Syndicate. Reprinted with permission. All rights reserved.

Differentiation develops to a variable degree during childhood through interactions between the individual and the emotional patterns in the family of origin. The patterns, in turn, derive from the previous generations. The key relationships for improving one's intellectual-emotional maturity are those with one's parents, because they hold the original, unresolved emotional fusion that influences all interactions. If adult children and their parents can get to know each other as people—relating with appropriate closeness but with less counterproductive emotionality—they can then relate more rationally with others.

Even as an adult, relating straightforwardly with one's parents is difficult. Relationships with members of the family of origin continue to be complicated. One-to-one relationships are stable when things are relatively calm. When anxiety increases, both parties behave in ways that draw a third party into an emotional triangle. A triangular arrangement can stabilize the relationship to some extent. Cross-generational triangles consisting of two parents and a child or one parent and two children seem to be the universal building blocks of family and individual dysfunction. The broader picture is one of multiple triangles interlacing in complex shifting arrays involving individuals outside the family, as well as the family members.

My Family Work

For 4 years I have been working on my own family issues, beginning by gathering facts about my family. The Bowen method uses the genogram (see Figure 9.1) to elicit and organize information (21–23). I am 39 years old, the sixth of seven children. Since I am 12 years younger than my next-oldest sibling, I grew up mainly as an oldest child, with a younger sister. [Bowen theory elaborates on Toman's work on sibling constellations (24).] My wife and I grew up in the same small town, and we have been married for 17 years. She was an oldest child, with a brother 7 years younger, and is a psychiatric social worker. We have a 7-year-old son and a 3-year-old daughter.

My father died in 1984 at the age of 83 from emphysema and heart failure. Despite having two operations for lumbosacral disk disease during his 50s, he continued to work as a bricklayer until retiring at age 75. In association with family turmoil each time, he had two duodenal ulcers. Until the past few years, he appeared to be relatively uninvolved with the family, seldom talking to any of us. He provided the main financial support, and built and fixed things for us. My father appeared to cope with the anxiety associated with closeness by distancing from us emotionally. The rest of the family interacted in ways that tended to keep him on the periphery.

My mother, 78 years old, has had high blood pressure and gallbladder problems. She prefers more emotional closeness than my father did, and

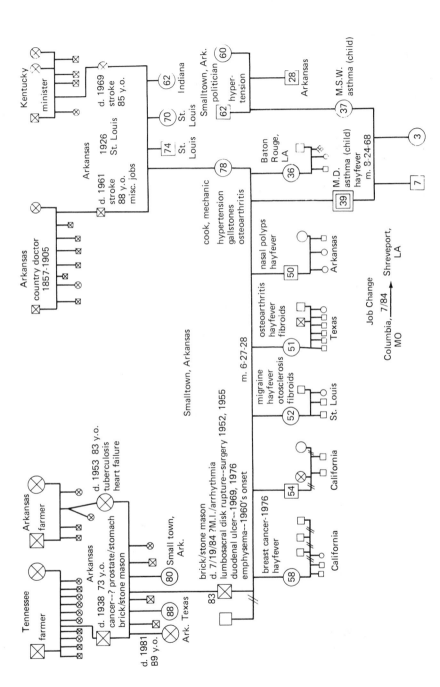

FIGURE 9.1.   The author's genogram.

has been somewhat overinvolved with several of us. She was very protective of me, which had advantages and disadvantages. She encouraged positive self-esteem with strong messages that I was cared for and special, and she encouraged a strong drive for achievement (typical for a mother of a doctor-to-be). During childhood her protection helped me feel secure, but during adolescence it felt intrusive and smothering.

My parents' relationship appeared to be a fairly distant one from my vantage point. They, like both sets of grandparents, seldom expressed affection verbally or physically. Combining both parents' patterns, I fluctuate between intense closeness to and considerable distance from others. When I am more anxious than usual, I tend to distance from family or work, depending on the source of the anxiety. In this respect, going for a run like the daddy in the cartoon can be a useful respite or an inappropriate escape.

My father was the fifth of eight children, the only one of four male children to survive to adulthood. My mother was the oldest of four children. My wife and I closely match my parents' sibling configurations, each having peer experience with the opposite sex, but having sibling rank positions that coincide. (My father and I were functional oldest male children, and my wife and mother were both oldest children.)

Advantages of coinciding ranks include understanding each other's mind set and having similar attitudes about taking responsibility. On the negative

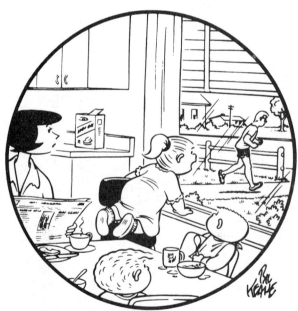

"I think maybe Daddy doesn't like it around
here. He's always runnin' away."

side, having the same sibling rank tends to generate counterproductive conflict; two oldests such as my wife and I have difficulty making a final decision on an issue where we do not agree. We may negotiate decisions with more difficulty than my parents did, partly due to recent shifts in societal norms for sex roles. In addition, since my mother-in-law has asserted herself with her husband more than my mother did, her parents shared major decisions more equally than my parents.

The main task of the work with my family has been to differentiate better from my parents by reducing the intensity of my triangular interactions with them. In addition to my primary emotional triangle with my parents, Figure 9.2 shows similar triangular relationships in past and present generations.

The basic features of my main family triangle are:

1. Marital relationships with considerable overt distance and underground intensity.
2. Mothers overly close to, and fathers distant from children.
3. Sporadic conflict within or between generations when emotional closeness increases too much for comfort.

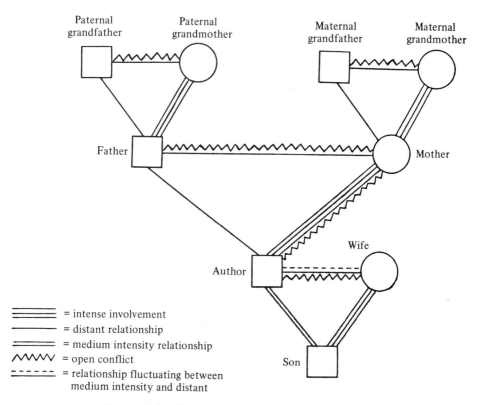

FIGURE 9.2.   Emotional triangles in author's family

Bowen Theory posits that getting to know each parent as a person dilutes entrenched emotional patterns and clears the way for choosing new preferred ways of behaving. I have talked extensively with my mother and father about their early lives, and understand them much better now. I was surprised to learn that my dad had served as the anesthetist for my home delivery by an old-style family physician, holding an ether-soaked rag near my mother's nose during the delivery.

I bridged some of the distance between me and my father by sharing my doubts and fears with him and soliciting his advice—new behavior for me. During the last 6 months of his life, I finally talked with him about my fear of death. He, in turn, talked, even joked about some aspects of dying. Since my family never talked about our feelings about death, this was a breakthrough.

For years we had enjoyed the cherries from a tree Dad planted in our yard and tended. While helping make the arrangements for my dad's funeral, I felt very sad, but also pleased, as my mother, younger sister, older brother, and I picked out a beautiful cherrywood casket. It was one of the few smooth cooperative efforts I can remember making with my family. Without planning to, I spoke at the graveside about my finally getting to know Dad, and about how hard it was to love and be loved by him.

After beginning to deal with my parents about death and dying, I can talk about these issues more comfortably with patients and families. Working with my family has helped much more than courses and seminars on death and dying. I have not resolved my own fear of dying, but have finally begun to accept the inevitability of my death, and the deaths of my patients.

With my mother I have begun to change a pattern of considering myself special and expecting to be treated accordingly. [This pattern appears to be nearly universal among physicians (10).] As one way of weakening this pattern, I now wash dishes and cook some when I visit home, instead of just letting my mother wait on me. During the time around my father's death, I discovered that I was really not as uniquely special to my mother as I had thought. She is very attached to all of us, and in some ways more so to some of my siblings than to me.

As part of developing an adult–adult relationship with my mother, I began to reveal myself by talking about work stresses and problems. Previously I hid problems from her, trying to look good no matter what, and I rejected her advice with an irritated response or withdrawal. Now that we have gotten to know each other better and I have dampened my reactivity, her comments feel supportive rather than intrusive.

It takes years to effect lasting changes in the ways one relates to others. To make a so-called second order change requires *being* different (thinking about oneself in a distinctly different way), not just *doing* something different (25). Redefining oneself with respect to family patterns is uncomfortable and, at times, depressing. It is unsettling to acknowledge that perpetuating certain lifelong attitudes and behaviors can create serious problems, and to admit that big-time change is necessary.

Influence on Patient Care

After working on my family issues for a year and a half, I concluded that some family patterns were blocking my *being* a complete physician. I grew up in a financially marginal working class family and still do not identify positively with some aspects of being a physician. I realized that I shared some of my father's cynicism about doctors. To become more comfortable thinking of myself as a physician, I have focused more on the healing and teaching roles that I can perform well and feel good about.

When caring for female patients, I am now more aware of my tendency to overfunction with them (to try to rescue them from their problems), and to try to take care of them emotionally like I thought my mother needed me to do for her. When I maintain an appropriate distance—caring without being fused—I think I encourage patient independence more genuinely. I was secretly flattered that many of my residency patients refused to see any of the other doctors, and would wait until I was available (sometimes inappropriately). I no longer need to have patients see me as so special, though I still enjoy being valued.

I can now predict from patients' genograms how I am likely to interact with them, based on my family patterns and theirs. Since I tend to distance from male authority figures and hostile women and tend to underfunction with them, I push myself to return calls from these kinds of patients and to follow up promptly on unfinished aspects of their care. My family work has influenced the intensity of some interactional tendencies. After working through much of my anger at my father and closing the distance between us while he went through the last stage of chronic obstructive pulmonary disease (COPD), I can deal more calmly and effectively with smokers and with COPD patients who continue to smoke.

I often realize during a patient visit that I am too close or too distant to be effective, and can sometimes become more objective and adjust my distance accordingly. Other times, I do not figure out what happened until afterward (e.g., while dictating the progress note). On these occasions I make mental and written notes about the dysfunctional dynamic and try to do better the next time. The following case example highlights the closeness–distance dynamic.

An attractive 42-year-old female, AB, presented in September, 1984 with chronic severe diffuse pain in her legs and low back of 2 years' duration. An extensive evaluation by another physician had turned up no evidence of disease in her nervous, musculoskeletal, or vascular system. She had quit working the previous year due to the discomfort. She also was not taking satisfactory care of her home and family. The history and normal physical examination gave the impression that serious disease of a predominantly organic nature was unlikely.

Mrs. B's husband had been married four times previously and had a history of excess alcohol intake. For about 3 years Mrs. B had been getting hostile letters and phone calls from an unknown person saying that her husband wanted to leave her. Mr. B denied knowing who this person was.

While seeing this patient, I consciously tried to avoid repeating my basic triangular pattern with this family. Considering my close maternal relationship and paternal distance, and the "damsel in distress" scenario, I could easily side with Mrs. B and try to rescue her from Mr. B. This would have been detrimental to the doctor–family relationship and the family's welfare. I realized this, and managed to stay reasonably neutral, enlisting the husband in the effort to figure out the meaning and function of the leg pain.

I did, however, repeat the intensity component of my pattern by pushing the patient to quickly see her problem the way I did. Not taking into full account the indications from her genogram that the family of origin was very poorly differentiated (multiple serious mental health problems), I quickly encouraged her to understand the leg pain as a symptom of unresolved conflicts. A colleague saw her and recommended that she go to Al-Anon to explore the alcohol issues in her family of origin and nuclear family.

Mrs. B was unable to deal with this forceful attack on her psychologic defenses against painful reality, and she decompensated into a psychotic state for several weeks. With medication and inpatient psychotherapy, her coping improved and she resumed her normal roles. Since that episode, I have seen her only once for routine care. Her defense mechanisms were restored and the underlying issues were still being avoided. I did not force the relationship issues again. If she requests more counseling in the future, I will proceed more slowly and cautiously, negotiating more limited goals with her.

As a clinician, working with my own family has impressed me with the usefulness of a multigenerational data base for understanding people's concerns and for helping them with their existing and potential health problems. I had previously done a skeletal genogram most of the time with new patients, and only occasionally expanded it very much. I now expand the skeletal genogram when it or the patient's presentation suggests the presence of important family factors. I inquire more often about aunts, uncles, cousins, nieces, and nephews, and try to get exact dates, rather than just the year of birth, marriage, and death.

Beginning early in residency training, I have done short-term, problem-oriented psychological counseling frequently as part of the comprehensive services I offer as a family physician. The family therapy training has allowed me to work with a few families at a time in more long-term counseling.

When beginning family-oriented counseling, during the first two visits I do a detailed three-generational genogram, which takes 60 minutes or more, including exploring some basic family dynamics (21,23,26). In doing multigenerational family counseling, the expanded genogram is the basic tool for evaluating the family and guiding the counseling.

The multigenerational perspective works well for counseling single family members or couples. I do not insist on seeing the whole family at one time, although having the whole family in at some point is often useful, and sometimes crucial. Systemic family change occurs through the change made by any individual in the family system. I work with the family member(s) who are most symptomatic or motivated to change. A major goal is to encourage someone to become a less anxious presence within the family and through their own change, to lead the family toward improved functioning (27). Some clinicians think that having most or all family members come in for a family counseling session is necessary to maximize the clinician's objectivity and opportunities for observing family interactions firsthand (see Chapter 7 for details). A busy physician will probably find it easier to work mostly with individuals and adult couples, except in the early stage of addressing the concerns of a child-focused family.

To encourage patients to discover for themselves the nature of their problems and potential solutions, I do less directive advising and ask more "systemic" questions (28). Except for severe acute problems, I schedule counseling visits less frequently (usually monthly now). With families who are interested in growth as well as improved coping, I focus more on improving general functioning.

Working with families in this way seems to be more practical than the frequent convening of whole families for weekly counseling. The multigenerational approach is complex enough, however, that many physicians will not want to use it or any other family therapy method as their main way of working with families therapeutically. Short-term, problem-oriented approaches such as those of Doherty and Baird are easier to learn and apply (29).

Regardless of the specific approach used, the clinician can profit from analyzing how his/her own family issues influence interactions with patients. Particularly when the doctor–patient relationship is unsatisfactory, it is often useful to ask oneself several questions:

1. How might my own family patterns be playing a part in what is going on?
2. How could I change my part of the interaction to avoid repeating my dysfunctional family pattern with this person?
3. What could I do differently in the future when I realize that a similar situation is threatening to develop into a problem?

Influence on Teaching

My major family pattern, the closeness and distance dialectic, applies to teaching as well as to patient care. Standing on firm emotional middle ground, I can make better contact with residents and medical students. Hospital work with seriously ill patients has been easier to do since talking with my father a lot while he was in the hospital. When he had severe respiratory distress, he no longer saw the hospital as a place to avoid, but rather as a haven.

Being aware of a tendency to overfunction with residents and medical students, I usually ask the residents systemic questions now instead of spoon-feeding them with canned answers and cookbook recipes. Because change comes slowly, this approach is difficult for learners who want behavioral skills that are easy to learn and apply. Cultivating the necessary forbearance to change entrenched patterns is also difficult for patients, who usually desire quick, painless solutions to their problems.

At times I encourage a resident who is having personal or professional problems to look at his/her own family issues to help understand the problems better, as in the example below.

In September, 1984 a male third-year resident headed the three-person family practice ward team while I was the attending faculty. Three times during the month, he became angry and verbally abused coworkers (an intern, a nurse, and a medical student). After I learned about each episode, I asked how it came about, stated that I considered the abusive behavior to be unprofessional and counterproductive, and encouraged him to find more acceptable ways to deal with anger. Checking with other staff members revealed a history of regular angry outbursts of this sort.

After the third episode, I did his genogram and discovered that both his parents were alcoholic. Furthermore, he had unilaterally ceased communicating with them several months ago. He was not aware how much his relationship with his parents was affecting his job performance and professional future, as well as his marriage. I suggested that he might benefit from some long-term therapy or counseling.

He began psychotherapy soon thereafter, focusing on issues with his parents. In the past 9 months his interactions with others have improved greatly, with only rare expressions of less intense ire directed at others or "the system." He has contributed numerous positive suggestions for improving the Family Practice Center. (He had previously been cynically critical.) In a subsequent survey of how courteous the residents are to staff members, he was rated average. After he had been out in practice for a few months, he commented that the anger issue was an even more important one for him to work on in that setting, since his long-term livelihood and happiness depended on satisfactory working relationships with many different people.

In the past I probably would have helped perpetuate the resident's dysfunctional pattern, either by avoiding dealing with him (like he was avoiding his parents), or by confronting him in the same hostile way he sometimes related with others.

Becoming aware of one's family patterns appears to be advantageous. How can physicians integrate this kind of awareness into their busy lives as practitioners out in the community? Medical school and residency training are probably the most opportune times to begin learning about how one's family can affect one's effectiveness as a physician. Family issues could be identified and worked on while learning about oneself and the doctor–patient relationship. Once out in practice, physicians with significant unresolved family issues would benefit from setting aside a regular therapy appointment with someone with whom they could work comfortably.

Influence on Administration

Being aware of my family patterns is also helpful in relating to coworkers. Preventing and managing conflict among clinic employees is probably the most difficult aspect of my being the clinic director. I suspect this is also true for many physicians out in community practice. I try to keep a medium distance with staff members that I supervise. The lessons from my family work prompt me to stay in touch with people routinely, which can prevent some problems.

When things get tense, I monitor my urges toward intense closeness or distance, and suppress my urges to engage in open conflict with someone (fight) or to go to the library (flight). Working closely with others to solve problems and manage conflict is uncomfortable. Choosing and sticking with a reasonable course of action, however, produces better results than perpetuating issues through avoidance or conflict.

With respect to relationships with colleagues, an awareness of my triangling tendencies is helpful. Alliances tend to form in reaction to situations in our department, as in all organizations. I try to observe the dynamics and respond to them rationally, while muting my emotional reactions to them. My goals are to maintain good working relationships with everyone in the department, and to avoid siding with my natural allies against likely adversaries.

Being an overvalued functional oldest child helped create a strong drive to excel. Due to career ambitions and my distancing tendency, I periodically get overinvolved with research and writing projects (such as this book). When too much energy goes to endeavors other than my family life and core job performance, both suffer from neglect. Ironically, in the academic world rewards such as tenure and professional reputation depend largely on scholarly output (research and writing), which must be squeezed in somehow without interfering too much with teaching, caring for patients, administrating, and family life.

Influence on Personal Life

One's time must somehow be allocated between professional activities and personal and family life. I am reminded of one of my medical school classmates who did a juggling act during which he gradually ate most of several pieces of fruit while he juggled them. The size and numbers of objects steadily dwindled as he juggled. Sometimes life feels like an inverse fruit salad juggling act, where one juggles objects that continually increase in size and number, while feeling that there is a stiff penalty for dropping anything. Many of us are reluctant to confront the fact that we control the number and size of the things we juggle. We are doing it to ourselves, and there is a price to pay for continuing unabated. Learning to say "No, thank you," and mean it, is a valuable survival skill.

In my nuclear family I am spending more time comfortably with my wife and children by monitoring my tendency to distance, and by thinking about the probable consequences of chronic distancing (emotional isolation and increased risk of having some kind of serious chronic illness). As part of feeling less entitled to having things my way, I also ask my wife and children more often how they would prefer to spend time together. I have not found permanent solutions to the perpetual dilemmas of balancing medicine and the rest of life, but my current provisional strategies seem more compatible with avowed long-term goals and priorities, and the results feel better most of the time.

Learning Exercise #1: Thinking about Your Family Patterns

Study your own genogram with the following questions in mind:

1. What are the patterns of illness and dysfunction?
2. What are the implications of these patterns for your health, health habits, and life-style?
3. How could your family patterns affect your effectiveness as a physician?
4. What kinds of patients would you be most likely to have difficulty with? What kinds of difficulties? How could you minimize these difficulties?

How to Start Working On One's Own Family Issues

Here are some guidelines for working with one's own family. The key elements for getting started include:

1. Establishing a therapy relationship with someone who has made substantial progress with his/her own family issues and who can "coach" your efforts (ask you thought-provoking questions and give you relatively objective feedback and useful suggestions).
2. Regular contact with each member of the family of origin.
3. Gathering lots of facts about the family.
4. Observing and analyzing emotional process patterns.

The methods for making changes with respect to one's family patterns (not changing one's family) involve:

1. Going slowly (solid change takes years to consolidate).

2. Establishing one-to-one relationships with each family member that get away from counterproductive patterns of the past.
3. Becoming more objective about one's interactions with others.
4. Taking responsibility for changing only one's own part of interactions, not trying to change those of others.

Conclusions

Working on my own family issues has helped me improve my job satisfaction and performance as a clinician, teacher, and administrator. Working on family issues from another systems perspective, such as that of Satir (30), may yield similar benefits, but Bowen Family Systems Theory offers some advantages for biologic-minded clinicians who want to understand themselves and their patients better. The clinician who works on his/her own family issues can be more effective with patients who have problems that evoke touchy areas in the clinician's own family.

References

1. Velasco de Parra, ML: Changes in family structure after a renal transplant. Fam Proc 1982;21:194–202.
2. Ferrari M, Matthews WS, Barabas G: The family and the child with epilepsy. Fam Proc 1983;22:53–59.
3. Huygen FJA: Family Medicine: The Medical Life Histories of Families. Nijmegen, The Netherlands, Dekker and Van de Vegt, 1978.
4. Penn P: Coalitions and binding interactions in families with chronic illness. Fam Syst Med 1983;1(2):16–25.
5. Scheinberg M: The family and chronic illness: A treatment diary. Fam Syst Med 1983;1(2):26–36.
6. Steinglas P: The alcoholic family at home. Arch Gen Psychiatry 1981;38:578–584.
7. Velasco de Parra ML, Davila de Cortazar S, Covarrubias-Espinoza G: The adaptive pattern of families with a leukemic child. Fam Syst Med 1983;1(4):30–35.
8. Walker G: The pact: The caretaker–parent/ill child coalition in families with chronic illness. Fam Syst Med 1983;1(4):6–29.
9. White M: Anorexia nervosa: A transgenerational perspective. Fam Proc 1983;22:255–273.
10. Gerber L: Married to Their Careers: Career and Family Dilemmas in Doctors' Lives. New York, Tavistock Publications, 1983.
11. Glick ID, Borus JF: Marital and family therapy for troubled physicians and their families. JAMA 1984;251:1855–1858.
12. Christie-Seely J, Fernandez R, Paradis G, et al: The physician's family, in Christie-Seely J (ed): Working with Families in Primary Care: A Systems Approach to Health and Illness. New York, Praeger, 1984, pp 524–546.
13. Guerin P, Fogarty T: The family therapist's own family. Int J Psychiatry 1972;10:6–22.

14. Ferber A: Follow the paths with heart. Int J Psychiatry 1972;10:23–33.
15. Bowen M: Family Therapy in Clinical Practice. New York, Jason Aronson, 1978, pp 337–387, 461–547.
16. Kerr ME: Family systems theory and therapy, in Gurman AS, Krisken DP (eds): Handbook of Family Therapy. New York, Brunner/Mazel, 1981, pp 226–264.
17. MacLean PD: A Triune Concept of the Brain and Behavior. Toronto, University of Toronto Press, 1973.
18. Sagan C: The Dragons of Eden: Speculations on the Evolution of Human Intelligence. New York, Random House, 1979, pp 53–83.
19. Kerr ME: Cancer and the family emotional system, in Goldberg J (ed): The Psychotherapeutic Treatment of the Cancer Patient. New York, McMillan Free Press, 1981, pp 273–315.
20. Schmidt DD: Family determinants of disease: Depressed lymphocyte function following the loss of a spouse. Fam Syst Med 1983;1(1):33–39.
21. Titelman P: A family systems assessment profile: A schema based on Bowen Theory. The Family 1984;11(2):71–80.
22. Guerin PJ, Pendagast EG: Evaluation of family system and genogram, in Guerin PJ (ed): Family Therapy: Theory and Practice. New York, Gardner Press, 1976, pp 450–464.
23. Pendagast EG, Sherman CO: A guide to the genogram. The Family 1977;5(1):101–112.
24. Toman W: Family Constellation: Its Effects on Personality and Social Behavior, ed 3. New York, Springer, 1976.
25. Terkelsen KG: Toward a theory of the family life cycle. In Carter EA, McGoldrick M (eds): The Family Life Cycle: A Framework for Family Therapy. New York, Gardner Press, 1980, pp 35–44.
26. Kramer JR: Family Interfaces: Transgenerational Patterns. New York, Brunner/Mazel, 1985, pp 34–48.
27. Friedman EH: Generation to Generation: Family Process in Church and Synogogue. New York, Guilford Press, 1985, p 3.
28. Penn P: Circular questioning. Fam Proc 1982;21:267–280.
29. Doherty W, Baird MA: Family Therapy and Family Medicine: Toward the Primary Care of Families. New York, Guilford Press, 1983.
30. Nerin WF: Family Reconstruction: Long Day's Journey into Light. New York, Norton, 1986.

CHAPTER 10

Future Directions for Family-oriented Medical Care: Research, Education, and Practice

Michael A. Crouch and Janet Christie-Seely

Broad Questions for Research, Education, and Practice

Until recently the relationships between the family and health and illness had not been investigated scientifically. Clinicians have always dealt with family factors in various ways; they have had to do so because health and the family are inextricably interwoven. Just as ancient healers and 19th century horse-and-buggy doctors must have done, modern clinicians have responded to the family aspects of their patients' lives, mostly based on their intuition and own life experiences. Medical teachers have rarely tried to advise their students about how to handle such matters, since they lacked a scientific knowledge base on which to found educational precepts. Because research, teaching, and practice are interdependent, this chapter will attempt to glimpse into the future in all three areas, beginning with research.

Current Research

Researchers currently investigating family systems with respect to medical practice are trying to answer three broad questions whose answers have great import for the medical educator and the primary care clinician:

1. How do families affect the health and illness of their members?
2. How are families affected by their members' health problems?
3. How do families, health care providers and the health care system interact with each other?

Within each broad question many specific issues are being investigated, and some tentative answers have begun to emerge.

Families as Determinants of Health/Illness

Families are thought to influence the health of their members in two basic ways. Predispositions to illness are transmitted genetically from one generation to the next, and individuals adopt life-styles and health habits that their parents and other relatives model while they are growing up. Numerous common diseases and health problems show a consistent familial pattern, including coronary heart disease (1), peptic ulcer disease (2), anxiety disorder (3), and breast cancer (4). For a few conditions like familial heterozygous hypercholesterolemia, a clear-cut genetic component has been identified (5). For other familial conditions, such as Type I and II diabetes and alcoholism, although identical twin studies show a strong genetic component, the exact pathophysiologic mechanism is unidentified (6–8).

This discussion revives the old nature–nurture debate about the degree to which genetically transmitted characteristics and predispositions affect people's lives, compared to social learning and other life experiences (including family dynamics). Trying to answer this question definitively is futile because nature and nurture are as intertwined as mind and body are. It may be that family dynamics and other psychosocial factors are more rooted in genetically determined predispositions than is commonly appreciated (9,10).

Recent information suggesting that genetic predispositions strongly influence the patterns of social interaction in higher animals comes from recently reported primate research (11). Rhesus monkeys have a very consistent social organization, in which the adult males spend most of their time with other adult males, some time with their female mate, and only about 1% of their time interacting with their immature offspring. The mother, by contrast, spends a majority of her time with her young.

Newborn Rhesus monkeys who were kept apart from all adults and fed by a mechanical surrogate mother interacted with each other chaotically, lacking a clear social structure even after they had grown up and reproduced. After two generations of living only with other socially isolated peers, however, the third generation of offspring duplicated the normal pattern of social interaction described above. These observations strongly support the notion of a species-specific social organization in Rhesus monkeys.

Although human beings are arguably more complicated than Rhesus monkeys, the remarkable similarity of most human cultures around the world over long periods of time suggests that much of our social behavior is also affected by some genetic preconditioning. The discipline of sociobiology has analyzed animal and human behavior and arrived at similar controversial conclusions (9,10). Humans share many characteristics with other higher animals, including an innate protectiveness of living space (territoriality) and a strong tendency to interact with others of one's kind (socialization). Considering how humans resemble other animals can help the clinician understand anxious patients better.

Familial patterns can also reflect socialization more than heredity in some instances. Family researchers and clinicians have described how families pass down learned interactional tendencies from one generation to succeeding generations (transgenerational patterns) (12). Primate research also provides evidence that social learning can modify genetic influences (11).

Female Rhesus monkeys can be bred true for overreactivity to stimuli ("anxiousness"). Such "up-tight" females do not parent their first offspring competently; they neglect or abuse the firstborn about 80% of the time. Less reactive (calm or "laid back") females can also be bred true; they parent firstborn offspring much more adequately, feeding and protecting them diligently. If female offspring of anxious mothers are placed with calm foster mothers, the offspring are much more calm when grown than when parented by anxious mothers. More importantly, they parent their firstborn offspring much more competently. If offspring of calm mothers are raised by anxious foster mothers, they remain relatively calm and are competent mothers when mature despite being parented by anxious mothers.

In the situations above, favorable nurture overrides unfavorable nature, and favorable nature overrides unfavorable nurture—in other words, if either nature or nurture is favorable, the outcome is positive. In humans, the destructive power of inadequate nurturing seems much greater, probably due to the longer period of human dependency, and the greater complexity of human social learning and emotional makeup.

One of the rediscoveries of the 1970s was a growing awareness of the potency of psychosocial stresses as contributors to illness. Stress often affects health adversely, as discussed in previous chapters. Adequate social and family support can buffer individuals against becoming ill when they are subjected to stress. In a recent longitudinal controlled study, researchers tried to bolster social support in individuals with low social support and high stress levels (13). During the 6-month follow-up period, the intervention group experienced significantly fewer illness days than the control group, despite no demonstrable improvement in their level of social support. These findings suggest that current methods for measuring protective aspects of social support may not be very sensitive or valid.

Effects of Illness on Families

Many illnesses affect the entire family. Widmer and Cadoret's research on depressed patients in a private family practice showed that other family members had more symptoms for 6 months prior to the patient's depression being diagnosed, particularly infections, pain, and functional complaints (14). The incidence of symptoms in other family members decreased markedly after the index patient's depression was diagnosed and treated (15).

The family can be affected by illness in many ways. The complexities of illness effects are seen in Steinglas' home observations of alcoholic families, discussed in Chapter 6 (16). This study sheds light on how alcoholic behavior recurs and is maintained. The secondary gains are appreciable for some family members, and the risks of change appear great to members of an alcoholic family system. The family system may support drinking behavior partly because family members feel more comfortable when the alcoholic member is drinking, despite their being opposed to the drinking in principle. This partly explains why it is so difficult to get an alcoholic's family to confront him/her with the problem directly and consistently support his/her getting the needed help.

The home observations also revealed a factor that was associated with whether or not offspring of the alcoholic showed signs of becoming alcoholic themselves (17). Alcoholic families can handle family rituals in one of two ways. They can carry on with family rituals, such as the opening of Christmas presents, as planned, whether or not the alcoholic is able to participate at the usual time (early Christmas morning, for example). Alternatively, they can incorporate the drinking into the family ritual by delaying the opening of presents until the alcoholic member sobers up. Offspring of alcoholics in the study appeared more likely to become alcoholic themselves if family rituals accommodate to the drinking, rather than being well maintained despite the alcoholism. Using this and the results of future research, clinicians may be able to give spouses and children of alcoholics more useful advice about how to reduce the risk of other family members becoming alcoholic.

Primate research has also demonstrated the effects of health problems on family interactions (11). In a Rhesus monkey colony a young male badly burned his hands on a power line. The family and colony as a whole refused to allow researchers to remove him for treatment, and they successfully cared for him themselves. For several days during the acute injury period, the father radically shifted his usual time allocation (1% for parenting) and spent about half of his time attending to the injured young one, splitting time with the mother. As the wounds healed, he gradually reduced his involvement, returning to his normal fathering time when convalescence was completed. Humans show similar crisis responses, with uninvolved males often becoming unusually involved in emergency situations, then reverting to their usual emotional distance when the emergency is over, or when it changes to a more long-term crisis (e.g., a child with leukemia).

Researchers at George Washington University are examining what happens over the long term with families of renal dialysis patients (18). One of their preliminary findings runs counter to the hypothesis that strong family support would be associated both with better compliance with medical management and with longer survival. Although the patients with more cohesive families did comply better with medical management, more of them died sooner than the patients with less cohesive families. One way of making sense of these results is to hypothesize that a member of a well-functioning family tends to live only as long as the quality of life is acceptable to the individual and to the family. In such a family, it may be that family members can die in a timely way when their quality of life is no longer acceptable, or when the family resources are being drained excessively by the ill member's continued existence. Another perspective would be that a member of a dysfunctional family has more "unfinished business" with other members; hanging onto life could provide more chances to work through difficult issues to some degree. Illness may also serve to stabilize the family homeostasis; this "tertiary gain" for the family, in concert with the secondary gain for the individual patient, may perpetuate or worsen chronic illness much more often than clinicians suspect (19).

Family Interactions with Health Care Providers

Some recent work describes how patients and family physicians relate to each other regarding family matters. Although most individuals would ideally like to get substantial help for family problems from their family doctors, they do not expect to receive much help. Three-fourths of the patients in one study thought that family matters were an appropriate focus for the family doctor's interest and were comfortable discussing them with their doctor, while one-fourth thought such discussion was inappropriate and were uncomfortable with talking about family matters with a doctor (20). Most patients thought the physicians in the study were quite interested in finding out about their family situation despite the physicians' spending relatively little time discussing family matters during these routine first visits with new patients. Apparently the patients were so unaccustomed to having a physician ask about their families that they were very positively impressed by the attention these physicians did give to family matters.

The above study also revealed problems with the way the physicians elicited family information and used it to help the patients. The physicians asked mostly closed-end questions (answerable with yes/no, or one of only a few choices, such as better/worse, good/bad). This closed style resulted in a physician-dominated interview; the patients were given few opportunities to reveal details about their concerns or their lives that related to why they came to see the doctor. The physicians did not make good use of the family information they did receive; they seldom followed up on a family history of hypertension, for example, by doing appropriate patient education about salt intake, exercise, and weight control (21). In another study, family history of serious health problems like coronary artery disease, diabetes, hypertension, and alcoholism was seldom recorded on patients' problem lists, where it could remind the physician to educate patients about the advisability of making life-style changes to avoid familial diseases (22). Apparently even among family physicians, who tend to get more family information than other specialists, there is considerable room for improving the way the family context is taken into account when caring for patients.

Future Research Directions

Family research in general is undergoing a turbulent adolescence. Several competing theoretical frameworks make sense intuitively and thus have reasonable face validity. When family assessment instruments based on different theories are compared, however, the results are confusing and difficult to interpret (23–26). Recent opinion favors using multiple measurement methodologies in any large study of family matters, to compare various models and facets of family functioning (27).

Scientific investigation of family-centered medical care is in its infancy. Several methods are currently being evaluated for obtaining a basic family data base that would give the physician the most information for a reasonable expenditure of effort and time. The genogram now appears to be the most practical method for the primary care physician to get accurate family information quickly. Predictive validity studies of the skeletal genogram and the expanded genogram are needed to assess their long-term utility, as are studies using the genogram in groups such as the elderly, minorities, and immigrants.

Cost-effective interventions to help patients prevent and deal with family problems are being developed and tested. Key research questions in this area include:

- How can the clinician best identify family issues and problems?
- When and how does a family issue become a family problem?
- What effects do family problems have on individual family members' health?
- What kind of interventions can prevent family problems from impairing the health of family members?

For many familial health problems, key contributing factors include behaviors that are learned in the family of origin, such as overeating and sedentary life-style. Through these health habits genetically predisposed people become obese, and in turn, hypertensive and diabetic in some instances. High dietary intake of saturated fat and cholesterol worsens matters, leading to hypercholesterolemia, atherosclerosis, and coronary heart disease. Little is known about when and how to intervene effectively with families to decrease the chance of individuals developing conditions for which they are at risk.

Research could also shed light on how to teach family-centered care to physicians, medical students and other health professionals. If family-centered care can be shown to be cost-effective, or just more effective than regular individual-oriented care, it would be easier to encourage its practice. Research could be done in private practice settings on how to integrate family-centered care into a financially solvent practice, and this information would, in turn, be helpful in teaching programs.

Research Methodologies for Studying the Family and Health

Medical researchers rarely regard qualitative and quantitative data equally, even when they gather both kinds of information. The quantitative data are regarded as more solid, and are thus presented confidently. Qualitative data, on the other hand, are apologetically presented as "anecdotal" or "impressionistic," if they are mentioned at all. Although medical science has made important gains by lumping together the experiences of many individuals with a disease, numerous breakthroughs have also been triggered by key observations of one or a few patients. It is still true today that observant, curious physicians can learn the most from their best teachers—their patients (28).

More work is needed that correlates direct observations of individuals and families with self-report and other-report measures. Medical scientists strongly prefer data collected by supposedly objective observations by the researcher. For many health issues this type of data is clearly desirable (e.g., blood cholesterol), but in research and clinical practice, observations formerly made only by the physician are now augmented by patient self-observations (e.g., home monitoring of ovulation timing by fluctuations in urine hormone levels, and measurement of blood pressure and blood glucose).

In the future, methods may be available for clinicians and researchers to more easily observe and analyze family interactions in the home. Although it seems far-fetched, sophisticated families in the future may be able to use advanced technology such as videocassette recorders, laser video disks, and home computer programs to observe and modify their own interactions, without ever contacting a physician or therapist.

Physicians may have gone to an unwise extreme in their allegiance to empirical science "by the numbers." In trying to avoid placing false trust in atypical individual data, the subjective baby can be thrown out with the biased bath water. Researchers who hope to discover the full underlying meanings of family matters and health problems may need to reassess the values that lie behind the terms "hard" and "soft" data.

Ethical problems arise when doing family research. The researcher may have difficulty maintaining the role of impartial observer and disinterested party. Families who have sustained contact with researchers may begin to see them as therapists or friends. The researchers may begin to feel involved with the family and have urges to help them with problems they are having. There is also the risk of exploiting families for the researchers' ends by encouraging dependency or continuing the study against the best interests of some families.

Despite the considerable obstacles to research on the family and health and illness, major progress has been made recently. Investigators who are also clinicians are shedding more light on how to better understand the complex relationships and on how to help patients and their families more effectively.

Implications for Medical Practice

The authors believe that, besides helping their patients be healthier, physicians who use systems approaches routinely may conserve both their time and the patient's or society's money in the long run. Working with family matters at one point in time creates ripple effects down the line that, interacting with other influences, can help people improve their health and their lives. For example, a doctor advises a patient three times over a 5-year period to stop smoking because of his family history of emphysema and heart disease. The patient acknowledges each time that he should stop, but does not make a serious attempt to quit until his father gets lung cancer. Some individuals will stop smoking in response to just the father's illness, but others will continue unless additionally encouraged by their physician and other significant people in their lives (e.g., young children).

Most patients appreciate their physician's showing interest in their family (20). Such interest opens communication beyond the conventional bounds of the disease-oriented medical interview. Inquiring about the family improves doctor–patient rapport, and helps build the trust that is essential for a therapeutic relationship. An opportune time to tell patients about the family emphasis is when they first enter the practice. An introductory brochure, written at a sixth to eighth grade reading level in a noncondescending manner, could include the philosophy of care and range of family services offered by the practice. The physician can verbally reinforce these points and solicit questions about them during the first visit with each family member. Alternatively, interviewing each new family all together at once could yield more accurate family history information in less time than multiple individual interviews would take. Family interactions would be observed directly, and the family orientation of the practice would be communicated symbolically, as well as explicitly in words, during such an intake interview. With this precedent, subsequent family meetings around health and illness issues would be easier to convene.

The physician who includes detailed family information in the routine data base gets a broad perspective that fosters open-ended clinical reasoning and decision making. Additional information suggests more hypotheses to be considered and tested during ongoing management. The family physician who works with the patient's family context will take better care of many patients than if the family context were neglected.

The office setting establishes the tone for the physician's practice. The following features encourage family-centered care (29):

- A waiting room that:
  - is large enough to comfortably seat patients and accompanying family members or friends;
  - is furnished and decorated in colors, textures, and styles that are warm and "homey";
  - has paintings, drawings, photographs, or prints of family life on the walls;
  - includes a play area for young children, with books and toys;
  - has a bulletin board with pictures of the babies and children in the practice;
  - has a bulletin board with information and notices about family health resources, classes, seminars, programs, news items;
  - has a supply of free materials—pamphlets, flyers, etc.—on common problems with family overtones (e.g., sex, contraception, seat belts, depression, alcoholism, abuse, suicide).
- Some examination rooms large enough for the physician, the patient, and two to three other family members to all sit down during regular visits;
- One comfortably furnished family/counseling room where eight to 10 people can sit for an hour or more for a family or group meeting, counseling, or patient education. If this room is devoted to only these purposes during office hours, it will be used more for patient meetings than if the room is used for multiple purposes (staff lounge, library, etc.).

Practice management decisions can also promote family-centered care. Since such care often takes more time in the short run, realistic expectations may be established for desired daily patient volume with this consideration clearly in mind. From observing and talking with family physicians in private practice, a daily average of 20–30 patients in 8 hours seems conducive to good-quality, comprehensive family-centered care and modest financial success. Some family physicians see 60 or more patients a day. Under these circumstances, the physician's focus necessarily shifts away from comprehensive holistic care to a narrow, complaint-oriented practice style that seems likely to be both unsatisfying for the physician and unsatisfactory to the patient in the long run.

Physicians may encourage care for all family members by arranging discounted office visit fees for multiple family members when the additional members can be taken care of quickly (two siblings with mild sore throats for $5–10 each after the patient with a severe pharyngitis has been seen for $15–25, for example). Many physicians now either see "piggybacks" free, or see them only for a full office fee; neither of these approaches seem fair to both the doctor and the family.

A potential solution to the time crunch involved with spending time talking with patients about family and other psychosocial matters is to hire someone to do this as their main function in the practice—a social worker, psychologist, or trained counselor. Family physicians have reported this to be a valuable addition to their practice, with multiple benefits for the physician and patients (30).

The pros and cons of various schemes for keeping medical records in a family-oriented way have not been well studied. Because existing approaches such as family folders require substantial extra work for the physician and/or records personnel, for minimum short-term gain and unclear long-term advantage, few family physicians keep family-oriented records. Creative physicians may develop new ways to manage patient records in family-oriented systems that work better than the arrangements proposed to date (31,32).

If the physician maintains problem-oriented records, a family orientation would be reflected by having family-related entries on the problem lists more often than is the usual tendency (22). Recording family history items on the permanent problem list can remind the physician to keep them in mind and to follow up on them during visits for other purposes. Some family-related problems worthy of being entered on the problem list include:

- Actual or potential problems in the nuclear family:
  - marital dissatisfaction, discord, separation, divorce, remarriage, joint child custody;
  - substance abuse;
  - violence or sexual abuse;
  - serious illness or death of a family member;
  - financial problems, including unemployment or underemployment.
- Problems with extended family:
  - intrusiveness or detachment;
  - serious illness;
  - institutionalization (nursing home placement);
  - losses (geographic separation, death).
- Problems of family with relationship to society:
  - legal problems, jail;
  - isolation from previous or potential social network;
  - serious dissatisfaction with neighborhood or neighbors.

The family physician may not be able to help the patient directly with many of these problems, but being aware of the family's unresolved issues will help assess and manage illness in its broad context.

The data base that is routinely gathered on each patient could include basic information about the family. Most commercial questionnaires do not elicit family data satisfactorily. A locally designed supplemental form can fill in the gaps, or the physician may wish to develop entire initial and interval history forms and have them printed locally.

The genogram (family tree) can be a very useful standard part of the medical record (33–36). The information on the genogram is most valuable if it is placed at or near the front of the medical record so that it is readily accessible during a routine visit. A xeroxed copy of the original genogram can be placed in each family member's chart, or if the family folder used and is brought out for all visits by any family member, the original genogram can be kept in the folder. The Family APGAR may prove to be a useful general screening tool for dissatisfaction with family life, and could be included in individuals' records at intervals for baseline and subsequent comparisons (37).

New technology will soon make it possible to gather physiologic data much more easily. Noninvasive methods are now available for measuring cardiovascular variables like total systemic peripheral resistance and stroke volume index (38). Besides revolutionizing the management of hypertension and coronary heart disease, these techniques could be used to measure patients' physiologic responses to their families in the office or at home. Invaluable information about stress coping and ways to manage psychophysiologic conditions like migraine may be obtained by monitoring various organ systems in the future.

For family physicians who have special interest in counseling families with problems, several approaches have been described that could be used with variable amounts of extra training at some point in the physician's education. A recent book of case discussions describes how clinicians may work with families on several levels, depending on their interest and training (39). Problem-oriented, crisis-oriented approaches work well for many situations (40,41). For patients whose health problems are closely tied in with emotional patterns running through several generations of their families (most patients, in the authors' experience), multigenerational family systems theory offers a cohesive framework grounded in biology. For growth-oriented counseling, the multigenerational approaches of Bowen, Satir, and Christie-Seely hold significant advantages for the experienced family physician who does advanced counseling with selected patients (42–46).

Family medicine is fostering a more egalitarian relationship between doctor and patient, but many physicians will still fall into a built-in rescuer response if they do not work to recognize and minimize this counterproductive pattern. When patients are encouraged to think and feel that they have choices in their own health care and in their lives as a whole, they are more likely to avoid being helpless victims, stuck in the secondary gain and reinforcing expectations of ill health. If the physician can help patients take risks to open up communication in their relationships and try new behaviors, the patients' self-esteem can increase and they can grow healthier. The physician can help patients learn from illness or negative relationships by pointing out that illness and unhappiness are often signs that the person or the family are stuck in a dysfunctional way of living.

Going beyond physical symptoms to the meaning of an illness may point out a lack of meaning in patient's lives. Frankl observed that the survivors of the Holocaust had a strong sense that their lives had meaning (47). Physicians rarely explore their patients' sense of purpose and meaning for their lives, perhaps because it raises doubts and discomfort about one's own satisfaction with life's meaning and purpose.

Another dimension related to health is a person's sense of control of his/her life. Feeling that one's life is out of control appears to lower resistance to a variety of illnesses and risk factors, such as obesity. A sense of being ruled by fate or chance also contributes to poor control of chronic illnesses like diabetes and hypertension. The issues of meaning and control are especially relevant when caring for depressed and anxious patients, and terminally ill patients.

A growth model of health care, as opposed to a hierarchical model, facilitates teamwork between physicians and other health professionals. People communicate more congruently in an egalitarian, nonhierarchical system that tends to enhance everyone's self-esteem. Being congruent (being oneself and being at ease with oneself) is as healthy for the caregiver as it is for the patient.

Educational Implications

As discussed in Chapter 9, any clinician may benefit from examining his/ her own family issues closely over an extended period of time (48). During the past 10 years, appreciation has grown of the importance of professional self-awareness for managing chronic and acute stress, to facilitate self-fulfillment, and to prevent personal impairment and burnout (49). In the future, educational experiences that look at the emotional and illness patterns in one's family of origin may become more common in the training of health professionals, particularly in medical schools (50) and in residency training programs in family practice (51) and psychiatry.

Family-centered care offers the academic physician skills for better diagnosing and treating physical illness, as well as the opportunity to develop a special area of expertise that would tie in to numerous other academic areas. Family assessment skills could be taught as part of medical interviewing, clinical reasoning, and record keeping. Discussions of the doctor–patient relationship could be enriched by considering the family backgrounds of actual or hypothetical patients and the student physicians respectively, and examining the various kinds of interactions between those background issues. One educational approach that combines two desirable goals—learning about family systems and broadening the typically narrow education of the medical student—is to learn about families by reading the writings of keen observers of human behavior such as James Joyce, D.H. Lawrence, James Baldwin, and John Updyke (52).

In primary care residency training, gathering family data and responding therapeutically to family information and problems could be taught more systematically. Applying current knowledge and integrating new knowledge could breathe life into the biopsychosocial model of Engel (53,54). The biologic and psychosocial spheres could be integrated into many learning experiences so that most physicians would learn to pay attention to families and other social systems in ways that would help them better understand patients and help with their problems.

By cultivating an awareness of the family aspects of health and illness, clinicians will take better care of themselves and their own families, as well as their patients/clients and their families. Paying more attention to families will increase clinicians' abilities to prevent and manage illness and promote wellness. Working with families toward better health holds rich rewards for health professionals in the future.

Summary

The authors believe that understanding families is more useful than categorizing them into diagnostic pigeonholes labeled with either individual psychopathologies or family theory typologies. Physicians can learn more from the families they care for than they can ever teach them (28). The physician who learns well can take advantage of the occasional opportunities to help families discover more about themselves. If medicine is thought of as a meal, most clinicians would probably regard traditional biomedicine as the meat, with psychosocial and family matters regarded as the green vegetables—theoretically desirable, but less vital and less appetizing. A growing number of clinicians consider working with families to be both their daily bread and the spice that adds zest to medical practice.

References

1. Oscherwitz M, Krasnoff SO, Moretti L, Syme L: The relationship of myocardial infarction to parental mortality and longevity. J Chron Dis 1968;21:341–348.
2. Evans DAP: Genetic factors in the etiology of duodenal ulcer. Gastroenterol 1961;40:371–378.
3. Crowe RR, Pauls DL, Slymen DJ, Noyes R: A family study of anxiety neurosis. Arch Gen Psychiatry 1980;37:77–79.
4. Kelly PT: Breast cancer in the family: Not always risky. Med World News, June 23, 1980, pp 41, 43.
5. Brown MS, Goldstein JL: Familial hypercholesterolemia: A genetic defect in the low-density lipoprotein receptor. N Engl J Med 1976;294:1386.
6. Simpson NE: Diabetes in the families of diabetics. Can Med Assoc J 1968;98:527–532.
7. Goodwin D: Is Alcoholism Hereditary? New York, Oxford University Press, 1976.
8. Tattersall RB, Pyke DA: Diabetes in identical twins. Lancet 1972;2:1120–1125.
9. Wilson E: Sociobiology: The Abridged Edition. Cambridge, MA, Belknap Press of Harvard University Press, 1980.

10. Barash D: The Whisperings Within. New York, Harper and Row, 1979.
11. Suomi S: Lessons from animal models. Paper presented at the Conference on Research on the Family System in Family Medicine, San Antonio, Texas, January 14, 1985.
12. Kramer JR: Family Interfaces: Transgenerational Patterns. New York, Brunner/Mazel, 1985.
13. Blake RL: Social support and utilization of medical care. J Fam Pract 1980;11:810.
14. Widmer R, Cadoret RJ: Depression in primary care: Changes in patterns of patient visits and complaints during a developing depression. J Fam Pract 1978;7:293.
15. Cadoret RJ, Widmer RB, North C: Depression in family practice: Long-term prognosis and somatic complaints. J Fam Pract 1980;10:625–629.
16. Steinglas PA: A life history model of the alcoholic family. Fam Process 1980;19(3):211–226.
17. Steinglas PA: Alcohol and the family system. Paper presented at the Conference on Research on the Family System in Family Medicine, San Antonio, Texas, January 15, 1985.
18. Reiss D, McGee D, Yano K: Psychosocial processes and general susceptibility to chronic disease. Am J Epidemiol 1984;119:356–370.
19. Dansak DA: On the tertiary gain of illness. Comp Psychiatry 1973;14:523.
20. Crouch MA, McCauley J: Family awareness demonstrated by family practice residents: Physician behavior and patient opinions. J Fam Pract 1985;20:281–284.
21. Crouch MA, McCauley J: Interviewing style and response to family information by family practice residents. Fam Med 1986;18:15–18.
22. Crouch MA, Thiedke C: Documentation of family health history in the outpatient medical record. J Fam Pract 1986;22:169–174.
23. Green RG, Kolevzon MS, Vosler NR: The Beavers-Timberlawn model of family competence and the circumplex model of family adaptability and cohesion: Separate, but equal? Fam Process 1985;24:385.
24. Bilbro TL, Dreyer AS: A methodological study of a measure of family cohesion. Fam Process 1981;20:419–427.
25. Bloom BL: A factor analysis of self-report measures of family functioning. Fam Process 1985;24:225–239.
26. Sigafoos A, Reiss D, Rich J, Douglas E: Pragmatics in the measurement of family functioning: An interpretive framework for methodology. Fam Process 1985;24:189–203.
27. Fisher L, Kokes RF, Ransom DC, Phillips SL, Rudd P: Alternative strategies for creating "relational" family data. Fam Process 1985;24:213–224.
28. Barnett L: Barnacles, ballast, and balance. Fam Med 1985;17:265–169.
29. Crouch MA: Family-oriented care, in Robertson D (ed): Textbook of Family Medicine. Chicago, Year Book Medical Publishers (in Press).
30. Glenn ML, Atkins L, Singer R: Integrating a family therapist into a family medical practice. Fam Syst Med 1984;2(2):137–145.
31. Ruth DH, Rigden S, Brunworth D: An integrated family-oriented problem-oriented medical record. J Fam Pract 1979;8:1179–1184.
32. Shapiro DM: A family data base for the family oriented medical record. J Fam Pract 1981;13:881–887.

33. Jolly W, Froom J, Rosen MG: The genogram. J Fam Pract 1980;10:251.
34. Rogers J, Durkin M: The semi-structured genogram interview: I. Protocol. II. Evaluation. Fam Syst Med 1984;2(2):176–187.
35. Mullins HC: Collecting and recording family data: The genogram, in Christie-Seely J (ed): Working with Families in Primary Care. New York, Praeger, 1984, pp 179–191.
36. McGoldrick M, Gerson R: Genograms in family assessment. New York, Norton, 1986.
37. Smilkstein G, Ashworth C, Montano D: Validity and reliability of the Family APGAR as a test of family function. J Fam Pract 1982;15:303–311.
38. Eliot RS: Overview: Family systems, stress and the endocrine system. Paper presented at the Conference on Research on the Family System in Family Medicine, San Antonio, Texas, January 15, 1985.
39. Doherty WJ, Baird MA: Cases in family-centered medical care. New York, Guilford Press, 1986.
40. Doherty WJ, Baird MA: Family therapy and family medicine. New York, Guilford Press, 1983.
41. Sawa R: Family Dynamics for Physicians: A Guide to Assessment and Treatment. Lewiston, NY, Edward Mellen Press, 1985.
42. Bowen M: Family Therapy in Clinical Practice. New York, Jason Aronson, 1982.
43. Kerr ME: Family systems theory and therapy, in Gurman A (ed): Handbook of Family Therapy. New York, Brunner/Mazel, 1981.
44. Satir V: Peoplemaking. Palo Alto, CA, Science and Behavior Books, 1972.
45. Christie-Seely J (ed): Working with Families in Primary Care. New York, Brunner/Mazel, 1984.
46. Nerin WF: Family Reconstruction: Long Day's Journey into Light. New York, Norton, 1986.
47. Frankl V: Man's Search for Meaning: An Introduction to Logotherapy. Translated by Ilse Lasch. Boston, Beacon Press, 1959.
48. Crouch MA: Working with one's own family: Another path to professional development. Fam Med 1986;18:93–98.
49. Gerber L: Married to Their Careers: Career and Family Dilemmas in Doctors' Lives. New York, Tavistock Publications, 1984.
50. Association of American Medical Colleges: Physicians for the twenty-first century—the GPEP Report. Report of the Panel on the General Professional Education of the Physician and College Preparation for Medicine. Washington, DC, Association of American Medical Colleges, 1984.
51. STFM Task Force on Training Residents for the Future: Training residents for the future: Final draft report. Fam Med 1986;18:29–37.
52. Maccio ME, Garcia-Shelton L: Family medicine and literature: A natural match. Fam Syst Med 1985;3(1):27–33.
53. Engel G: The need for a new medical model: A challenge for biomedicine. Science 1977;196:129.
54. Like R, Reeb KG: Clinical hypothesis testing in family practice: A biopsychosocial perspective. J Fam Pract 1984;19:517–523.

Appendix A: Some Residency Training Programs Emphasizing Family Systems

Family Practice

University of South Alabama School of Medicine, Mobile, Alabama
Valley Medical Center, Fresno, California
University of California Irvine School of Medicine, Irvine, California
Santa Rosa Community Hospital, Santa Rosa, California (affiliated with the University of California at San Francisco School of Medicine)
University of Calgary School of Medicine, Calgary, Alberta, Canada
Mount Sinai Hospital, Toronto, Ontario, Canada
University of Connecticut School of Medicine, Farmington, Connecticut
University of Florida School of Medicine, Gainesville, Florida
University of Miami School of Medicine, Miami, Florida
University of Kansas School of Medicine, Wesley Family Practice Residency Program, Wichita, Kansas
Louisiana State University School of Medicine in Shreveport, Shreveport, Louisiana
University of Massachusetts School of Medicine, Worcester, Massachusetts
Michigan State University School of Medicine, East Lansing, Michigan
University of Michigan School of Medicine, Ann Arbor, Michigan
Hennepin County Medical Center, Minneapolis, Minnesota
University of Missouri School of Medicine, Columbia, Missouri
Montefiore Medical Center, Bronx, New York
University of Rochester School of Medicine, Rochester, New York
University of North Carolina at Asheville, Asheville, North Carolina
Case Western Reserve University School of Medicine, Cleveland, Ohio
University of Oklahoma Health Sciences Center, Oklahoma City, Oklahoma
Brown University School of Medicine, Memorial Hospital, Pawtucket, Rhode Island
Medical University of South Carolina, Charleston, South Carolina

Psychiatry

Medical College of Georgia, Augusta, Georgia
*University of Maryland School of Medicine, Baltimore, Maryland
Harvard Medical School, Cambridge Hospital, Cambridge, Massachusetts
*Massachusetts Mental Health Center, Boston, Massachusetts
Rutgers Medical School, Piscataway, New Jersey
*University of New Mexico School of Medicine, Albuquerque, New
    Mexico
*Albany Medical College, Albany, New York
*Albert Einstein College of Medicine, New York, New York
Division of Family Programs, Department of Psychiatry, University of
    Rochester, Rochester, New York
*Western Psychiatric Institute and Clinic, Pittsburg, Pennsylvania
*Texas Research Institute of Mental Sciences, Houston, Texas
Medical College of Wisconsin, Milwaukee, Wisconsin

---

*Requires over 400 hours of family therapy training according to survey reported
in Family Process (1981;20:147–54).

Appendix B: Some Family Therapy Training Programs, Centers, and Resources*

Organizations

American Association for Marriage and Family Therapy Commission on Accreditation for Marriage and Family Therapy Education, 924 West Ninth, Upland, California 91786

American Family Therapy Association, 1815 H Street, N.W., Suite 1000, Washington, D.C. 20006

American Association of Marriage and Family Therapy, 1717 K Street, N.W., Suite 407, Washington, D.C. 20006

Training Programs and Centers

Family Therapy Institute of Berkeley, Berkeley, California
Family Therapy Institute of Southern California, Los Angeles, California
Los Angeles Family Institute, Los Angeles, California
Center for Human Communication, Los Gatos, California
The Kempler Institute, Mesa, California
Mental Research Institute, Palo Alto, California
San Diego Family Institute, University of California San Diego, San Diego, California
Family Therapy Center Association, San Francisco, California
Family Therapy Institute of Marin, San Rafael, California
Bristol Hospital, Bristol, Connecticut
University of Connecticut, School of Family Studies, Storrs, Connecticut
Family Therapy Institute of Washington, Washington, D.C.
Georgetown University Family Center, Washington, D.C. (Bowen)

---

*This partial list was compiled by reviewing past volumes of Family Process and Family Systems Medicine, from suggestions by knowledgable family therapists, and from a listing in Family Process (1981;20:133–146). Numerous training programs exist besides these.

Family Institute of Chicago, Chicago, Illinois
The Depot, Chicago, Illinois
Purdue University, Department of Child Development and Family Studies, West Lafayette, Indiana
Menninger Foundation Family Therapy Training Program for Community Practitioners, Topeka, Kansas (eclectic) and Prairie Village, Kansas (Bowen)
Family Therapy Institute of New Orleans, New Orleans, Louisiana
Boston Family Institute, Boston, Massachusetts
Family Institute of Cambridge, Department of Psychiatry, Cambridge Hospital, Cambridge, Massachusetts
Kantor Family Institute, Cambridge, Massachusetts
New England Center for Study of the Family, Newton Centre, Massachusetts
Cape & Islands Family Institute, Pocasset, Massachusetts
Ann Arbor Center for Family Research and Training, Ann Arbor, Michigan
Family Therapy Institute of St. Louis, St. Louis, Missouri
New Jersey Center for Family Studies, Chatham, New Jersey
Canterbury Group Family Institute, Great Neck, New York
Family Institute of Westchester, Mt. Vernon, New York
Center for Family Learning, New Rochelle, New York
Ackerman Institute for Family Therapy, New York, New York (strategic)
Family Therapy Training Program, Division of Family Programs, Department of Psychiatry, University of Rochester, Rochester, New York
Southeast Institute, Chapel Hill, North Carolina
Family Institute of Cincinnati, Cincinnati, Ohio
Eastern Pennsylvania Psychiatric Institute, Philadelphia, Pennsylvania
Family Institute of Philadelphia, Philadelphia, Pennsylvania
Hahnemann Medical College, Department of Mental Health Sciences, Philadelphia, Pennsylvania
Philadelphia Child Guidance Clinic, Philadelphia, Pennsylvania (structural)
Galveston Family Institute and Center for Family Studies, Galveston, Texas
Houston Family Institute, Houston, Texas
Texas Tech University, Department of Human Development and Family Studies, Lubbock, Texas
Trinity Counseling Services, Princeton, New Jersey
Family Therapy Institute, Alexandria, Virginia
Center for Family Services, Blacksburg, Virginia
University of Wisconsin, Department of Psychiatry
Brief Family Therapy Center, Milwaukee, Wisconsin

Appendix C: Family Systems Research Programs/Centers

Mental Research Institute, Palo Alto, California (Haley)

University of California at San Francisco, San Francisco (Ransom)

George Washington University Department of Psychiatry, Washington, D.C. (Reiss)

Family Therapy Center, Washington, D.C. (Steinglass)

Peckham Experiment Network, Janet Bunbury, Watertown, Massachusetts

University of Minnesota Department of Family Studies, Minneapolis, Minnesota (McCubbin)

University of Minnesota, Division of Family Studies, Minneapolis, Minnesota (Olson)

Ackerman Institute of Family Therapy, New York, New York (Penn, Papp)

Division of Family Programs, Department of Psychiatry, University of Rochester, Rochester, New York (Lyman Wynne, Duncan Stanton, Robert Cole, Susan McDaniel, Judith Landau-Stanton, Thomas Campbell)

University of Oklahoma Department of Family Medicine (Ramsey, Stein, Patterson, Baird, Baker)

Philadelphia Child Guidance Clinic, Philadelphia, Pennsylvania (Fishman)

John F. Kennedy Family Research Center, George Peabody College, Nashville, Tennessee

Southwest Family Institute, Dallas, Texas (Beavers)

Wallingford Wellness Project, University of Washington, School of Social Work, Seattle, Washington

Appendix D: Some Family Systems Journals

The Family, Center for Family Learning, 10 Hanford Avenue, New Rochelle, New York 10805 (semiannual; Eileen Pendagast, Editor; $12/yr)

Family Process, Family Process, Inc., 149 East 78th Street, New York, New York 10021 (quarterly; Carlos Sluzki, M.D., Editor; $24/yr)

Family Relations, National Council on Family Relations, 1901 West County Road B, Suite 147, Saint Paul, Minnesota 55113 (quarterly; Michael Sporakowski, Ph.D., Editor; comes with membership in the National Council of Family Relations)

Family Systems Medicine, Brunner/Mazel, Inc., 19 Union Square West, New York, New York 10003 (quarterly; Donald Bloch, Ph.D., Editor; $28/yr)

Family Therapy Networker, 7703 13th Street, N.W., Washington, D.C. 20012 (bimonthly; Richard Simon, Editor; $15/yr)

Journal of Marital and Family Therapy, American Association for Marriage and Family Therapy, 1717 K Street, N.W., Suite 407, Washington, D.C. 20006 (quarterly)

Journal of Marriage and the Family, National Council on Family Relations, 1901 West County Road B, Suite 147, Saint Paul, Minnesota 55113 (quarterly; Jetse Sprey, Editor; comes with membership in the National Council on Family Relations)

Working Together: A Collaborative Health Care Newsletter, 137 Ferry Street, P.O. Box 250, Everett, MA 02149 (quarterly; Michael Glenn, M.D., Editor; $15/yr)

Appendix E: Suggested Further Reading about Family Systems and Health

Christie-Seely J (ed): Working with Families in Primary Care: A Systems Approach to Health and Illness. New York, Brunner/Mazel, 1984.

Doherty WJ, Baird MA: Family Therapy and Family Medicine. New York; Guilford Press, 1983.

Doherty WJ, Baird MA: Cases in Family-Centered Medical Care. New York; Guilford Press, 1986.

Gerber L: Married to Their Careers: Career and Family Dilemmas in Doctors' Lives. New York; Tavistock Pubs, 1983.

McGoldrick M, Gerson R: Genograms in Family Assessment. New York; Norton, 1986.

Nerin WF: Family Reconstruction: Long Day's Journey into Light. New York; Norton, 1986.

Sawa R: Family Dynamics for Physicians: A Guide to Assessment and Treatment. Lewiston, NY; Edward Mellen, 1985.

Simon FB, Stierlin H, Wynne LC: The Language of Family Therapy: A Systemic Vocabulary and Sourcebook. New York; Family Process Press, 1985.

Glossary of Terms

ABC-X model—a theoretical model for explaining how individuals and families deal with stress. (Hill)

Alliance—a relationship between two members of a system. This term, like coalition, is used inconsistently in writings about the family. (*See coalition.*) Structural family therapists use alliance to describe positive one-to-one relationships in families (e.g., parental alliance).

Autonomy—well-defined self, with capability of functioning independently with regard to important life decisions.

Biopsychosocial model—an expansion of the traditional biomedical model of health and illness to include the important psychosocial factors that are inextricably interwoven with the biomedical factors. This model emphasizes the importance of the physician's understanding the whole person in the context of the family of origin, the nuclear family, the extended family, the friendship network, the spiritual orientation, the workplace, the neighborhood, the community, and the culture. All of these spheres influence the individual's health, and any of them may be relevant to providing optimal care for the patient and family at some point. (Engel)

Boundary—an abstract family systems concept that refers to the unspoken rules governing how members of a system relate to each other and to the rest of the world. The clarity of a boundary refers to how emotionally involved the individuals are with each other:

1. Overinvolved, with little autonomy (diffuse boundaries).
2. Solidly connected with well-developed autonomy (clear boundaries).
3. Emotionally distant or cut off, with pseudoautonomy (rigid boundaries). (Minuchin)

Bowen theory—a family systems theory that postulates that an effective way to understand and work with individuals and families clinically is to gather detailed information about several generations of the family. This information is used to help family members understand the emotional patterns they are repeating from past generations, and to help them change how they relate to their family of origin and how they conduct their lives. Key clinical parameters are the level of differentiation and the level of anxiety in the family system. (Bowen)

Circumplex model—a typological classification of families derived from interrelating two continua (cohesiveness and stability); based on extensive research with nonclinical families. (Olson)

Coalition—a relationship between two members of a system. The term is used differently by various writers and clinicians. It is sometimes used to describe an overly intense dyadic relationship, which may be oriented against another member or members of the system (us-against-him/her/them). Coalitions may be transient or stable, functional (e.g., spousal) or dysfunctional (parent–child against the other parent).

Countertransference—the clinician's emotional response to, and fantasies about, the patient and family, derived from feelings and fantasies about the clinician's early caretakers. It can be positive (overvaluing and overtreating dependent patients who idealize the clinician), or negative (undervaluing or rejecting disliked patients who cannot be cured or who do not comply with the clinician's recommendations). (Freud)

Detouring—rerouting of conflict between two members toward a third member of a system in a overprotective (enabling) or accusatory (scapegoating) manner. The third member, often a child, usually develops symptoms eventually—recurrent headaches, abdominal pain, alcohol abuse, etc.

Differentiation of self—the degree to which one has established one's own values, life goals, and emotionally mature ways of relating to others. Well-differentiated individuals and families integrate rational and emotional functioning harmoniously and make sound life decisions even when anxiety and stress are increased. The important decisions of less well-differentiated persons and families are excessively influenced by strong emotional urges, especially when anxiety is increased. (Bowen)

Disengagement—extreme emotional distance in a relationship. Both parties are unable to sustain a closer relationship after the preceding closeness produced an intolerable level of anxiety. Thought of by structuralists as diffuse relationship boundaries and rigid individual boundaries.

Double bind—a contradictory communication that is repeated over and over such that the recipients of the message feel they have no viable choice (e.g., "change/don't change").

Emotional connectedness/relatedness—sharing emotional closeness with other persons. A healthy amount of connectedness involves relating in a clear, direct way around issues of mutual concern, while maintaining individual autonomy. Members of a relationship system get more anxious when the connectedness is closer or farther than they can comfortably tolerate.

Emotional cutoff—roughly synonymous with disengagement. The cool or cold appearance of emotional cutoff is thought to disguise a relationship that has been and continues to be very intense—so intense that extreme distance is necessary for both parties to control their anxiety and for them to survive. Major unresolved conflict underlies emotional cutoff. (Bowen)

Enabling—a process whereby one or more members of a system consistently shelter one member from experiencing the natural and logical consequences of his/her actions. Thought to be one of the basic processes that promotes substance abuse in a susceptible individual.

Enmeshment—a system process in which members are overly involved emotionally and lack individual autonomy. Family boundaries with the outside world are rigid and internal subsystem and individual boundaries are too diffuse. Individuals tend to overreact to any changes in each other's behavior, especially when their anxiety is up. (Minuchin) Roughly synonymous with Bowen's terms "emotional fusion" and "undifferentiated ego mass."

Ethos—thoughts and feelings that characterize a culture, including shared attitudes, beliefs, values, and understandings about how life should be lived, and about the nature of the world. The ethos of mainstream American medicine, emphasizing mastery and aggressive individual initiative, often conflicts with the cultural emphases of patients, who might, for example, subordinate self to family, or who may have a more fatalistic attitude toward sickness and death.

Executive subsystem—the relationship of members of the family responsible for making decisions, allocating resources, and rearing children. Usually involves one or more adults as parents. Children can be opted into this subsystem easily in single-parent families. An only child is also more likely to become part of the executive subsystem.

Explanatory model—a framework of thought by which each participant in a clinical encounter (clinician, patient, family member) tries to understand an episode in terms of its personal and cultural meanings. Most physicians explain illness in terms of the biomedical model. Key components of an explanatory model are notions about cause, timing of the symptom onset, pathophysiology (what's messed up and how), and the expected course and outcome of the illness. (Kleinman)

Extended family—members of one's family of origin (parents, siblings), family of ascent (grandparents, uncles, aunts, cousins, etc.), or family of descent (grandchildren, nephews, nieces, etc.)

Family Adaptation Adjustment Response—a theoretical framework for explaining how individuals and families deal with life, particularly with stressful events, situations, and relationships. (McCubbin and Patterson)

Family APGAR—a five-question, self-administered questionnaire that can be used to screen for individual dissatisfaction with five aspects of family life—availability of help (Adaptation), talking over problems (Partnership), acceptance and support of new individual activities (Growth), expression of and response to emotions (Affection), and sharing of time together (Resolve). (Smilkstein)

Family atomosphere—enduring, though changing, themes in a family. The atmosphere is a distillation of past experiences and related memories into beliefs, both factual and mythical, about family members and the family as a whole. Themes include health and illness beliefs, family mood, secrets, committment, and esteem.

Family Circle—a technique for having individual family members portray the interrelated emotional relationships in the family system by drawing small circles at various distances from each other within or outside a large circle on a piece of paper. (Thrower)

Family dynamics—a general term for the ways in which family members think, feel, and interact with each other and the world.

Family functioning—the patterns of interaction between family members, and the way the family as a whole tries to accomplish the day-to-day and long-term tasks of life. Major content areas of functioning include the meeting of physical and emotional survival needs, solving problems, making decisions, and dealing with conflict. Health habits, self-care practices, and utilization of the health care system are facets of functioning. The main processes of functioning are verbal and nonverbal communication for affective and instrumental purposes.

Family myth—a belief, shared to a variable degree by most or all family members, weakly based in their interpretation of some factual past history. Belief in the myth maintains a certain inner family image and generally allows the family to avoid dealing with difficult issues, such as taking responsibility for directing one's life to the extent possible, risking failure or success, handling sustained intimacy, etc.

Family of origin—the family grouping(s) in which an adult was raised, most often consisting of parents and siblings, and sometimes grandparents, aunts, uncles, etc. who lived in the home for some time.

Family of procreation—the family grouping in which an adult currently lives, most often including a spouse or partner and, at sometime during the life cycle in many families, children, grandchildren, and great-grandchildren.

Family-oriented counseling—helping individual family members or the whole family by such straightforward approaches as providing support in time of crisis, reassuring that particular feelings and behavior are normal given the situation, exploring the implications of various choices being considered, and suggesting other options the family has not considered. Family counseling may be done by seeing one member, a couple, a parent and a child, any subset of the family, or the entire nuclear family, and it may at times include members of the extended family, especially the family of origin or descendents (a grandmother, mother, and grandchild, for example).

Family secret—an event or situation that family members avoid talking about or dealing with openly because of their anxiety about it. The secret may be shared between some family members, and kept from others. Although the content of the secret usually consists of emotionally intense material involving sexuality or death, the process of communication about the secret is more revealing of family dynamics than is the content of the secret.

Family structure—the members of a family and how they are organized with respect to power or authority and emotional closeness. The characterization of boundaries summarizes fundamental dynamics of a family. (Minuchin)

Family systems theory—a theoretical framework that attempts to explain how individuals and families function in terms of circular, nonlinear interrelatedness, rather than in terms of linear causality. There is no *one* family systems theory; rather, there are a number of different theories, some of which share conceptual similarities disguised by semantic differences. Most theories also are tied, albeit sometimes loosely, to a set of clinical strategies and techniques intended to effect desired changes with families that ask for help, or who are thought to be in need of help for perceived actual or potential problems. Some theories include features of "general systems theory" such as homeostasis, feedback loops, and morphogenesis.

Family therapy—compared to family-oriented counseling, family therapy tends to involve more complex assessments and interventions. Family therapy is indicated more for families with more difficult and long-standing problems and with a lower baseline level of functioning prior to the development of the problems for which they are being seen.

Feedback loop—a process that promotes (positive) or reduces (negative) deviation in a system. Information reentering at a point in the system increases or decreases subsequent change in the system.

Fusion—roughly synonymous with enmeshment. Fusion is more often applied to overinvolvement between two members of a system, and enmeshment is more often used to describe a system as a whole. (Bowen)

Genogram—a diagram of the members and relationships of multiple generations of a family (family tree). (Bowen, Jolly, Mullins)

Group fantasy—shared and mutually shaped fantasies about what it feels like to be a member of some group (case conference, profession, nation) at a particular time. The fantasy is often out of the awareness of group members, but nonetheless mobilizes members, shaping the direction of group action. In a medical case conference, in addition to the official diagnostic and treatment agenda a shared unconscious agenda might be: "We're going to get this troll off our backs." (deMause)

Homeostasis—the tendency to maintain a dynamic equilibrium, minimizing overall change in the face of external perturbations and internal changes.

Joining—forming a therapeutic alliance with the patient, each individual family member, and the family as a whole.

Legacy—expectations by members of one generation of certain or all members of succeeding generations. The expectations are accepted to differing degrees by the heirs. (Borzormenyi-Nagy)

Mission—a special task assigned by a member of one generation to a member of a succeeding generation, to be done for the sake of the whole family. Missions are specific legacies that often involve accomplishment (or failure), caretaking, and immigration.

Morphogenesis—the tendency to evolve in substantial ways ("grow" in psychological terms) in response to external and internal changes, contributing to family vitality through innovation and enhancement. (Speer, *Family Process* 1970;9:259)

Morphostasis—processes maintaining the stability of a system despite external and internal changes. Morphogenesis and morphostasis describe a paradoxical dynamic of living systems; both types of processes are necessary for survival of a system for its optimal natural course. (Speer)

Multigenerational family systems theory—a conceptual framework that seeks to identify problematic patterns of emotional processes that have been replicated in successive generations of the patient's family. The clinician then tries to help the family understand the patterns and to help interested family members change through modifying how they handle emotional issues. (*See Bowen theory.*) (Bowen, Kramer)

Mutuality—emotional connectedness between members of a system. It involves both convergence for relatedness and divergence for separate individual identities (differentiation).

Nuclear family—stereotypically, the family membes in a two-generational family of procreation—husband/father, wife/mother, and children.

Organizing metaphors—a constellation or condensation of cultural images or symbols used to simplify, unite, or characterize perceptions, often to facilitate action. Military metaphors present the doctor as a soldier fighting in the trenches with magic bullets against the enemies of death and disease.

Overfunctioning—actions reflective of emotional overinvolvement, insufficient regard for the autonomy of another, and diffuse boundaries. Many marriages display a pairing of an overfunctioning member with an underfunctioning member. (Bowen)

Overinvolvement—excessive emotional closeness (fusion) to the extent that rational functioning is seriously impaired, especially around toxic issues and when anxiety is increased for any reason.

Paradox—a communication that simultaneously is true and represents a sort of challenge to the individual or family to change a target behavior. A paradoxical statement either predicts that they cannot or will not change, or urges them to maintain the current behavior and avoid the risk involved in changing. (Selvini-Palazolli)

Positive reframing—restating a family problem in a way that points out the purposefulness of the problem as an attempted solution to another problem in the family (decreased libido in a wife as a way of avoiding putting more pressure on a stressed husband).

Projection—attributing one's own motives, feelings, impulses, or attitudes to another person, together with the sense of being the object, rather than the source, of the attributes that one believes to be originating with the other person. A physician who is angry with a patient may not acknowledge his/her own anger, but instead feel that the patient is angry at him/her. This process can, understandably, eventually generate in the patient the very emotion originally attributed to him/her as the patient responds to the anger of the physician.

Scapegoating—the process of diverting conflict between two members of a system toward a third member in an accusatory way ("It's all his fault").

Shaman—one who claims the knowledge and power to master a group's mysteries and dangers. Most group members believe the shaman can allay their fears and anxieties by controlling the unknown forces. The shaman is the historic prototype and ancestor of all "medicine men" and modern physicians. In Mexican culture the shaman is called a curandero. Some black cultures in the United States still believe strongly in "root doctors" or "witch doctors." (La Barre)

Sociobiology—the scientific discipline that attempts to understand how genetically transmitted characteristics and predispositions influence the behavior of humans and other animals. (Wilson)

Strategic family therapy—an approach to family therapy that concentrates on the detailed processes of family functioning (communication) to assess a family's problems and to intervene therapeutically. This school of family therapy uses unorthodox counterintuitive interventions such as positive reframing and paradox. (Haley, Selvini-Palazzoli)

Structural family therapy—an approach to family therapy that emphasizes assessing family structure and intervening to change the structure in a way that allows the family to improve its functioning. (Minuchin)

Subsystem—an organization of relationships with functional significance within a larger system. Family subsystems include the marital, parental, and sibling subsystems. (Minuchin)

Triangle—three members of a system and their patterns of interaction. In many family systems, one of the three one-to-one relationships of a triangle appears overly intense (fused), with apparently positive closeness, and two of the relationships appear to be less positive, with cool distance and/or smoldering conflict. The primary triangle for most people consists of the individual and his/her mother and father. Patterns from this triangle are replicated later in life with one's spouse and children. (Bowen)

Underfunctioning—actions reflective of an insufficiently differentiated sense of self, and a low level of autonomy. Chronic underfunctioning is often associated with depression and various "physical" illnesses. (*See overfunctioning*.) (Bowen)

Working with families—being aware of the patient's family context, realizing how health and illness affect and are affected by family dynamics, detecting potential and actual family problems, and helping family members improve their mental and physical health by acknowledging

and dealing more effectively with their family dynamics. The clinician
can help the family by doing family-oriented counseling or family therapy
him/herself or by consulting or referring skillfully.

These definitions were written by the authors of this book. Several def-
initions were influenced by the material in Alvin H. Strelnick's article "A
Glossary" in *Family Systems Medicine* (1985;3(1):82–87). A source that
defines and discusses many family systems terms more extensively is *The
Language of Family Therapy: A Systemic Vocabulary and Sourcebook*
(New York; Family Process Press, 1985).

Subject Index

Index of Names